HEALTH HAVEN

PREVENTION AND RECOVERY FROM ILL HEALTH THROUGH THE USE OF ALTERNATIVE SOLUTIONS

DR MANJIT KAUR

Disclaimer

This book is designed to provide information and motivation to our readers. It is sold with the understanding that the author and publisher are not engaged to render any type of psychological, legal, or any other kind of professional advice. The content is the sole expression and opinion of its author. Neither the publisher nor the individual author(s) shall be liable for any physical, psychological, emotional, financial, or commercial damages, including, but not limited to, special, incidental, consequential or other damages. Our views and rights are the same: You are responsible for your own choices, actions, and results.

Published by DVG STAR PUBLISHING

www.dvgstar.com

ISBN: 1-912547-26-0
ISBN-13: 978-1-912547-26-5

DEDICATION

This book is dedicated to my patients, friends and family, especially my parents who inspired me to be where I am today.

CONTENTS

ACKNOWLEDGMENTS

My heartfelt thanks go out to my family as well as
all my patients who had faith in my treatments and trusted
me.
Thank you to all the people who gave me the opportunity to
work with their charities and made me humble.
I would like to thank Philip Chan who was my force of
inspiration and who mentored me throughout the book
journey.
I would also like to thank my publisher, Mayooran
Senthilmani, Labosshy Mayooran and the team at DVG
STAR Publishing for working with me to get my dream of
becoming a published author a reality.

FOREWORD

Is there simple solutions to complex problems, particularly in the area of Health? Hippocrates of Kos (c. 460 – c. 370 BCE), considered the "Father of modern medicine" gave the answer to that question long ago.

Prevention is better than cure!
It is said that: "An ounce of prevention is worth more than a ton of cure!"
One of the best cures is through the use of food combinations.

Who is Dr. Manjit Kaur?

She was born in Kenya. She brings a wealth of experience with her, and has studied in the UK and in four other continents, in Wholistic Medicine.

She is a skilled health practitioner, with qualifications in 9 therapies, and she has helped thousands of patients recover from a whole host of illnesses, even when her patients were given no hope by the NHS, other than surgery or chemo. She has been very successful in helping patients with blood sugar imbalances implement lifestyle changes and has been very successful in helping patients with IBD (irritable bowel disease), IBS (irritable bowel syndrome) and critical bowel conditions. These patients are living a healthy lifestyle without any surgical interventions.

Dr. Manjit has also been very successful in helping couples to conceive, with 90% success for women with PCOS (Polycystic ovary syndrome) or a history of Infertility in both male and females.

Worldwide, she is known as the Asian Media Host for Radio and TV shown over a 20 year period, as well as hosting four

TV Shows per week on Sky TV such as health shows, chat shows, vegetarian cookery shows and much more.

As a Philanthropist, Public Speaker, TV Presenter, Coach, Charity Award Winner, Sikh Sewadar Community Worker, Charity work is very close to Dr Manjit's Heart, she has funded a mammoth water irrigation project with the Bantu Tribe in Meru, Kenya working in high temperatures exceeding of 40 Celsius. This Bantu tribe is now successfully growing their own vegetable produce and also selling to the markets further afield.

Other projects includes setting up an Agave plant in the outskirts of Soroti in Uganda; helped widows in Punjab to open small businesses; guided and coached patients in drugs addiction centres also in Punjab. Her free acupuncture health camps in Italy and her community talk shows have given a wealth of knowledge to the congregation.

Dr. Manjit has a tireless, bouncing, energetic, charismatic personality.

She is dedicated to her patient's success until it is achieved. She has a warm friendly style in dealing with all her patients. In this book, Health Haven, Dr. Manjit will share with you some of her experiences and how to use the knowledge to safe guard you and your family's health.

Enjoy her book.
Good Health.

PHIIP CHAN
Award Winning Author of 10 Seconds Maths Expert and 10 Seconds To Child Genius.
International Award Winning Radio Host as seen on TV, Radio, Newspapers and Media.

Dear Readers,

Thank you for taking the first step to buy this book. This means you want to understand how to improve your lifestyle and learn how to deal with the struggles and stresses in your life, I am here to show you how to implement my unique branded solution that I have created in this book –Health Haven.

This book will certainly be a journey that will assist you and provide you with fundamental exercises that will help you to overcome situations, imbalances or ill health in your life. When times are difficult you will agree, we all need help and support and a listening ear. We all need someone to give us that comfort to overcome our struggles, and to give us a safe space where we can begin to tap into our innermost feelings, and sometimes we cannot relate with confidence until the right person walks into our lives. Whatever struggles you are currently going through, my aim is to help you to break away from the imbalance and give you the tools to use my Unique Branded System (UBS), which I have created in my clinic for patients to overcome their ill health, to implement food changes, rebalance their lifestyles, and to help them manifest their dreams and transcend their challenges
The challenge is there to excite us, give us confidence, and we get that triple effect from implementing these exercises and creating a better and healthier lifestyle.

When we are in a bubble of ill health we are locked up in shackles. Going in and out of hospital for allopathic treatments may not have given you the desired results, but I can passionately say that after practicing in my clinic, in my personal development and meditation, I've managed to direct an excellent skill set into practical application for patients to overcome their struggles and their frustrations.

Life is like a navigator and using the five step process you will be able to overcome the dark days of pain and struggle. By using this UBS, you can create massive changes and bring back your quality of life and wellness.

In this book I hope you will be able to regain strength and connect with your inner self and live a life which enables you to fulfil your dream.

Life is like an experimental journey, if we take the wrong routes we may not be able to reach our target. By seeking help and guidance about what has happened, we will be able to understand our journey and have a stronger connection to ourselves. We can unleash trapped feelings by using certain processes and communicating with our inner selves. I hope these chapters in this book help you develop the mindset and gratitude to rejoice life, and not regret the mistakes made along the journey.

In the UBS, all the techniques will give you ways forward and help you overcome challenges and reach your ultimate goal. In any illness, I understand there is apprehension, fear, sadness, anxiety, negativity, and lack of happiness. All the opportunities that come into our lives may look like huge tasks, but I hope that you will be able to grow and achieve your objectives in life, to use the tools provided to motivate you.

Life serves us lots of things on a golden plate, but it's taking the opportunity at the right time, and so few of us take the opportunity and plunge, and others may feel sorry and procrastinate.

I started my journey by learning the hard way, realising that I was not just cooking three meals a day for a large family; I had the desire to know a lot more about allopathic and alternative medicine.

Life was a struggle but I had to understand what my journey is about. I had to walk through life's trials and tribulations and not doubt my ability; I have learnt how to stay courageous and confident.

In our life's journey we need to find ourselves, achievable goals and liberate ourselves from our conscious and subconscious mind. We need to cultivate solid beliefs and thoughts, and we need to take responsibility in implementing the necessary changes to create a healthier life. We can delude ourselves and forget, a lot of people come into our lives that influence us and help us. They give us opportunities with their words of wisdom, but it doesn't serve us when we interact with them from our negative experiences and all of our negative thoughts. If implemented with positivity, wisdom can help us develop in to a better person.

We saw our parents charitable deeds throughout our lives and this made us humble. We knew we had to help the poor and needy. The projects that I took on were a dream and a vision, and my parents planted that seed. My father travelled in the 50's from Kenya with very little money, to the port of Mombasa from the port of Mumbai. With his talent in carpentry he started a new life and after three years of hard work, he saved up enough money to pay for my mother's and three year old elder sister's journey by ship which took twenty eight days, sailing through the rough seas of the Indian Ocean. Both parents reunited and settled happily in Nairobi. Over the years my parents were blessed with the birth of five healthy children.

Life was great in Kenya and we thrived on humble food and the food was made with love and my mother recited prayers and meditated whilst cooking which added the biggest spice! Although the food was simple, it was not depleted of minerals or vitamins and we looked very healthy and had vibrant energy. We were never fatigued or bored as we were so connected to mother earth, and our immune systems were so strong, compared to the children of today's generation.

We were happier and more successful in school as well. The strength we had all came through cultivating the correct mindset and the determination to seek opportunities to be the best in what we were doing.

We had a happy childhood. We even had the joy of eating apples and grapes which were an expensive commodity, with my parent's humble salary of fifteen pounds per month.

Celebrating several events in our religious festivals kept us connected with the community and as we embraced with friends from all walks of life and cultures we learnt to respect each person's beliefs and practice of their religion and we lived in harmony, and maintained respect for all.

Celebrating and uniting in diversity, by sharing and communicating certainly gave us a great structure in our early lives. I built a strong identity and developed positive communication skills throughout my educational life. Good food and juicing was something my mother always encouraged us to do. To this day I still embrace it. After studying Dr John Walker's raw food and juicing therapies, I introduced the food combining therapies in my Clinic and noticed a rapid recovery of my patients with combination of treatment, a healthier diet and supplementation.

Even in the warm country of Kenya, my mother always made sure we had two fish oil capsules a day and it took me twenty years to understand that what she did for us was right. Today cold pressed fish oils are highly recommended for general health and well-being.

Life can be exciting, but it is a journey where we have to find the balance with being determined and disciplined in our goals and stay true to our feelings and support and console those who need help. That's what I practiced in school and throughout my higher education and in my general life. I am very active in sports (badminton, hockey, tennis, and netball), it not only enabled me to thrive but also gave me the willpower to take challenges in life and achieve my goals. The feeling of rejoicing victory is most exhilarating when you have achieved your designated targets. True joy and happiness of having achieved our goal is celebrated when we apply the knowledge we have attained through life's experiences. When you use the same concept of willpower in any other life's situations that confront us in ill health or sickness, it should not be an overload to your mind but take it as a challenge to change and rebalance your body. Master the daily visualization and gratitude suggested in the book and this will optimise your full potential. By repeating the exercises you will improve your health and transform your life.

The golden nuggets that you will learn, will be an experience that will take you to success and give you more precious moments in life. It's what you are passionate about that you can share with the world and through transition and change of mindset, all these challenges will ignite you, empower you and teach you to become more powerful in your thought process. You'll be able to share your strengths to those who need it most and make them feel worthy so they can have their dreams and their withheld aspirations fulfilled.

My objective is to show the reader my techniques, to make them feel motivated and to give them the tools necessary to overcome all their health issues through the use of alternative supplements, diet, nutrition, bio energetic medicine, flower remedies, and the balance of the human body quantum field.

Sometimes we need to work on it. I liken life to a circus, where lots of different acts may be happening on the stage, and it can leave us feeling apprehensive, but like a clown in the show we need to create and keep humor in our lives!

Based on the wealth of knowledge, wisdom, understanding and reasoning, your actions will be converted into what you want in reality.

When you have the knowledge, you can transform your life experiences into positivity and have more inner strength to convey your passion to your friends and family. My dream became a reality when I believed deep inside, through my sports activities that I could make mammoth changes in the tasks I was doing although they seemed difficult. Eventually these obstacles became easier to shift.

You too, will go on to achieve your goals for the right reasons and understand that the situations in your life, that were once baggage and heavy to carry, will be much lighter, and you'll be able to accept yourself and begin to help others who have gone through a similar journey.

BY TUNING INTO YOUR SUBCONSCIOUS MIND, CONNECTING DEEPLY WITH YOUR HIGHER SELF, YOU WILL ACHIEVE YOUR DESIRED GOALS.

INTRODUCTION
DR. MANJIT'S LIFE JOURNEY INTO ALTERNATIVE & WHOLISTIC MEDICINE

I was born in Nairobi Kenya, and after my education in Kenya, I continued to study and widen my knowledge of the application of Holistic Medicine in the UK, Spain, Switzerland, Germany, USA, North and South India and in Beijing.

After my education, I started my own practice in Alternative and Holistic Medicine. Being devoted to spreading the knowledge of good health and being a great believer in "charity begins at home" as the proverb goes, I myself have proven that a human can stay very healthy by observing a few golden rules.

I am globally renowned for my TV and radio programs that were broadcasted across the world. I have been a practitioner for many years, and health has played a huge role during my whole life. Having fulfilled one of my ambitions of beginning to educate people on how to eat and live healthily, via my radio and television programs, I am now concentrating on my other aspirations; providing the world with healthier alternatives and bringing awareness of addiction and dangers of sugar which is one of the onsets of diabetes.

In my cook shows I have created recipes eliminating the use of table sugar and instead used alternative sugars and Agave Syrup .

In the two decades of me broadcasting on satellite TV and radio shows, I have brought awareness across the globe to my listeners. I have spoken about daily eating habits and how to support the body when it is diseased with foods, by presenting an alternative diet, provided solely from mother earth. Each of my programs are dedicated to a particular disease or function of the body, helping people improve the state of their organs by monitoring intake of fresh fruit and vegetable juices, not forgetting a daily routine of physical exercise.

The natural sugar in juicing recipes that I give each of my patients according to their pitta and kapha and the tri-dosha, (the Ayurvedic terms) help to enhance the body's healing processes. These raw juiced foods help to destroy and eliminate sugar blues and dips in energy throughout the day. They reduce craving and hunger pangs, as the live natural unsweetened juices are high in fibre and help cleanse the intestinal walls.

"Food and feeding are the most important aspects of a path to good health.". And I believe in treating a person with a "health and disease therapy".

My vast therapeutic knowledge and treatment of diseases afflicting the colon, eyes, ears, nose, tongue, throat, stomach, liver, pancreas and other organs of the body have brought relief to thousands of my patients who come from all over the world.

I have boundless energy and enthusiasm when it comes to maintaining a good healthy lifestyle, and practicing what I preach. This is also reflected in my three children. I have brought up my children with juicing in the morning and to use as much organic produce in their cooking as possible when making family meals whilst steering away from sugars, sweets and fast foods. I believe a child will follow what you practice, so good choice of foods and cooking nutritious organic meals have to be introduced from the time of weaning. The media and fast food industry is changing the taste buds of children who now crave for sugars, simple carbohydrates and fried foods.

Charity

In Meru, at the border of the Elsa game reserve in Kenya, I donated a complete water irrigation system for the local Bantu tribe who were dying of starvation because of drought in a remote rough terrain. Their crops were dependent on rain fall and seeing the damage of the drought of four years, I was very disturbed and profoundly touched by seeing the dying local people. I prolonged my stay, as there were no government long-term projects to help these natives. A water irrigation system complete with a reservoir was installed, which would store 40,000 litres water in case the river dried out.

A project was planned to pull water from a dangerous twenty five foot cliff to irrigate the land. Whilst everyone spent their Christmas 2005 with their families, I was with engineers installing the system in heat of over 40°C. The village was a nine hour drive through very muddy and very rough roads. My venture brought hope and dignity to people who are now growing and crop feeding 2000 local people and even selling the produce to the game lodges as far as 35km away.

Having organized six dinner and dance events which took over two months to organise hosting over 300 people each time raising money for the blind and needy and for Hemkunt children's education society. Large funds were also donated to institution for disabled children with polio.

Sadly in this Twenty First Century, it has been noted a lot of children are not eating a healthy balanced diet, which should include the five portions of essential fruits and vegetables a day, and which should have some starchy foods like whole meal bread, rice, brown pasta, potatoes, a variety of greens, and all colors of vegetables, some dairy, fresh and not processed cheese produce and alternatives such as almond, soya milk and hazelnut milk, and including legumes, pulses and the family of beans, with meat, fish and eggs and other proteins that are a good source of vitamin B12.

Variety in diet is what is essential for the body to grow and a good source of vitamins and minerals in a range of foods will optimize children's health and maintain good immune systems. I believe parents are a role model and have a very important role in helping children develop good healthy eating habits which will be their foundation and children are nurtured into these foods. They will have developed their taste buds to appreciate home cooked meals rather than processed, frozen and fast foods which are all beige and brown. I believe that in ten years' time young people's kitchen larders will be stored with processed and fast foods, and this is worrying to me.

It has been noted that some children have not tasted a raw carrot from the age of seven and are steering away from home cooked meals. I believe that in ten years' time, young peoples' homes will not even have a cooker to cook meals. Instead, there will be his and hers microwave cookers and larger and larger walk through freezers to store pre-cooked meals which contain huge amounts of fats, salts, sugars, colourings and preservatives.

With our Vitality and Rejuvenation Clinic now firmly established, I specialise in Colon Hydrotherapy and also offer over nine other treatments for a vast range of health problems. From day one, I have made people aware that the master organ of the body, the colon, has been subject to so much risk and damage in these modern, demanding times of ready meals and quick processed foods We are almost mutilating ourselves in the name of comfort and laziness.

My message is simple:

"Action must be taken before it is too late!"

Healthy, well balanced food consumed at the right time is crucial for a healthy body. The nutrients in a well-balanced diet keep your immune system strong and allows for the general development of your body. Freedom from sickness and disease is essential to your peace of mind as it allows you to focus on your physical activity. Whilst maintaining a balanced diet eating wholegrain, fruits and vegetables, it is important to cut back on bad fats, namely trans and saturated fats, and choose polyunsaturated and monosaturated fats. The benefits of good oils vs bad oils has been well established in the food industry, but sadly the use of trans fats and saturated fats is still very extensive.

I educate and guide people who listen to my health shows by creating food plans and advising changes in their lifestyle patterns. When these golden rules are followed religiously, the body will rebalance and replace the nutrient levels.

When the cells carry this nutrition in the bloodstream, the damaged and diseased organs begin to repair the cellular damage, thus improving the energy flow and the frequency with which the organ should be functioning.

"Life is very short"

Eye-opening observations by Dr. Manjit Kaur

Lifespan is being increased with surgical intervention, but diseases which were not occurring until the age of 60 plus are affecting people in their 20's and 30's. They are becoming victims of several illnesses due to food and lifestyle. Several examples are:

- Constipation; the root cause of all illness
- IBS (Irritable Bowel Syndrome)
- Heartburn
- Stomach aches
- Refluxes and burps
- Bloated ness and flatulence
- Sluggish digestion
- Gall bladder inflammation
- Liver imbalance and insulin resistant problems
- Stress
- Poor immune system
- Migraines and headaches
- Candida, thrush
- Low energy and fatigue
- Obesity
- Poor sleep
- Buildup of mucus and phlegm
- Allergies
- Fertility problems
- Joint aches and pains
- Low sex drive
- Poor circulation
- Poor vision
- Poor concentration
- Depression

- Eczema and skin allergies
- Parasite infestation

Weakened guts caused by consuming highly sweetened and salted foods, white flours, fried, frozen, canned and microwave foods are partially to blame. Gall bladder and liver problems lead to early onset of diabetes. Heart conditions and coronary artery blockages, water retention in the body, hypertension and skin conditions are conditions that are being accelerated in the general population by around twenty years!

Deep down inside, we all know that the most important thing in life is to feel good, maintain good weight and eat sensible well-balanced foods at the right time in a peaceful and happy state of mind.

But do we actually practice this?

We leave everything for tomorrow, we make resolutions, and keep bluffing our mind and body. Deep down mankind is weak and gives little to achieve personal wellbeing.

Good health can be maintained on a physiological and psychological level by relieving worries, easing anxiety and tension and instead replacing that with joy and laughter, which will increase feelings of positivity and abundance.
That is the pathway to a healthy and fulfilled life.

When running on high stress levels, over eating, drinking excess alcohol, smoking, and an over indulgence in high sugared foods, this can lead to a habitual nature, which over time will create a load on the digestive system and increase the risk of further stress, and malfunction of other vital organs. One indulgence leads on to another and that becomes the habitual nature of the individual.

We have entered the Twenty First Century so what is new or different? There is a higher sugar intake with a risk of diabetes now in every household. With more comfort in homes there is also more pain. Unhappy and unhealthy because of our mental flaws and being more educated yet more ignorant, has resulted our beautiful existence into one of anger, hatred, pride, jealousy, anxiety, selfishness, depression, and compulsive addictive behaviours with imbalanced mental thoughts; we ourselves are contributing to our own destruction and death.

The air we breathe and need to live has ironically turned poisonous, filled with toxic emissions from engines and machinery and CFC (chlorofluorocarbons) gases, causing free radical damage with depletion of the ozone layer in the atmosphere.

Mother earth has provided us with an abundance of herbs, roots, vegetables and fruits. Unfortunately, the farming industry has turned food into potential death-traps by using spray chemicals and pesticides to create larger quantities of produce, but in this process they have also destroyed the nutritional goodness.

My aim in writing this book is to bring awareness and a wealth of knowledge and understanding to my readers and help them to make sound choices in their diets, emphasising on reduction of "bad sugars", a healthier diet in general and a good lifestyle to integrate all these elements.

The body only declines in health when it has reached a cliff hanger of total organ intoxication. At this point, one or more organs of the body will start to malfunction causing cellular and molecular destruction. Major electrical impulses will stop transmitting between the brain and connective organs, causing a full blown illness.

Onset of disease is part of nature's effort to remove morbid matter, which attracts germs from the body cells flowing in the body. We need the curing properties of nature's five elements; sun, air, earth, water and fire. In my clinic, good nutrition plays a major role in alleviating how subdued our bodies have become due to invasive toxic painkillers, which disturb the stomach pH levels causing indigestion, oesophagus inflammation, liver overloads, and abdominal and gut problems.

Health is the physical state of the patient.
Harmony is the mental state of the patient.
Peace is the combination of spirit and healthy body.
A harmonious and peaceful mind is the definition of a
perfect human being.

Within my clinic, I observe the lifestyle choices of my patients to help them achieve a more rounded and healthy development of their personality via physical fitness, mental alertness, emotional balance and spiritual well-being. The choices we make regarding food, exercise and good rest are vital factors that help maintain the equilibrium of good health.

Eating more foods containing sugars causes addictive behavior patterns resulting in stress on the stomach, liver and pancreas. This forces the excess secretion of adrenaline by the adrenal glands, leading to glucose imbalance in the blood and thus can cause diabetes mellitus.

Stress, worry, germs, viruses, and low immune systems all trigger off disease as a result of the violation of the natural laws of health.

Behind every addiction be it sugar, alcohol, smoking, or drugs, is a "Trapped Mind". Free the mind and you are on the pathway to a full recovery after detox. To start the healing process and to prolong life, mankind has to free himself from addiction, reduce stress, negative thoughts and anger, hatred, fear, jealousy and greed. Before putting sugar coated and sugar ladened food into your mouth spare a thought to how badly you can suppress your body's immune system.

Think BEFORE you invade your body with deadly sugars.

"THOUGHTS FIRST COME TO THE MIND, ACTION FOLLOWS LATER".

Sugar contains no nutrients and is what is known as empty calories. Instead sow sweet positive images in your thought process and think of vibrant foods which will reflect on you attaining a healthy body.

The consequences of eating too much sugar

Those people who are eating too many wrong sugar containing foods will find that Kapha, which is one of the Ayurvedic forces is imbalanced.

Kapha is a force that makes lubrication (mucous) and structure (bones, muscles, fats joints, connective tissues etc.) of the body. People eating chocolates, sugar loaded foods, ice cream, and sweetened drinks etc., will find their Kapha percentage increasing in the body. With excess kapha one get symptoms of cough, asthma, excess mucous, congestion in the chest and obesity.

Sugars affect the mood regulating brain chemicals too. Abusing the body with addictive sugar may cause imbalances. These foods aggravate the deficiencies in serotonin levels resulting in a brain chemistry imbalance. This numbs the person to the work of the "feel good factor" of neurotransmitters. Naturally, this then makes it difficult to stay away from the sugar and addictive substances, and it creates a vicious cycle.

In the new millennium life style, the eating habits of people has totally changed. Life is fast and stressful and we are living under a toxic blanket of a polluted atmosphere and it is dramatically affecting the health of people. Diseases triggered by excess sugar in the diet namely diabetes, asthma (with mucous membranes of the lungs infected and inflamed) and skin conditions are very common in today's young generation

In my clinic, the technique of treating the patient in health and disease and diet therapy, plays a major role in rebalancing their malnourished bodies. By using food planning techniques linked to their Ayurvedic body types I bring awareness to the patient and make them more health conscious and nutrition minded.

We eat foods to generate fuel in our body. Pungent, bitter, and sour foods produce heat and some acts as coolants, but sugar produces bad heat and mucous.It takes years of abuse to degenerate the body and let disease step in. It takes half the time to repair, regenerate and rebalance again.

Educating the patient to prevent disease by making modifications in their daily food intake can dramatically change the state of their well-being. Some other guidelines are given to patients:

☑ Eat according to your bodies' needs and requirements
☑ Never cook in anger because the food will not be energized
☑ Using spice is cooking with "LOVE"
☑ Practice simplicity in cooking
☑ The stomach cannot cope with too many varieties of food in one meal
☑ Never over eat , always leave some room in your stomach

☑ Use the right fats in cooking
☑ Eat more organic and natural foods free from pesticides, chemicals, fertilisers and sprays
☑ Avoid saturated fats
☑ Never over cook your food
☑ Avoid foods with sugar or sweetened with artificial sweeteners
☑ Reduce salt in your cooking
☑ Have more seasonal foods from the country you live in
☑ Reduce red meat
☑ Introduce more organic fruits and vegetables
☑ Don't forget your greens for the day
☑ Reduce wheat and yeast ladened products
☑ Avoid white floured breads and pastries
☑ Have a varied diet in your daily eating routine. Too much of the same food without change causes food allergies
☑ Allow time for the stomach to digest the last meal before eating or snacking again (minimum 4 hours break)
☑ Too much overload into the stomach slows digestion
☑ You must take a conscious effort to chew your food
☑ Avoid talking and chewing at the same time
☑ Never eat in anger and haste
☑ Always eat in a peaceful harmonious environment
☑ Always sit down and eat away from the T.V and computer
☑ Avoid fluids with your meals, have one hour after a meal
☑ You must relax for 20 minutes after a meal
☑ You must drink at least 3 litres of water a day
☑ Avoid too many pre-cooked meals
☑ Look out for artificial colours and preservatives in foods
☑ Never eat late. Your last meal should be 3 hours

before bedtime
- ☑ Remember if calories in is not calories out, body mass and fat increases around your abdomen, buttocks and thighs
- ☑ Regular exercise is vital

In my clinic, good nutrition plays a major role in maintaining a good state of health.

Remember sugar is stored as "FAT".

Eating sugary foods from an early age increases the chance for sugar addiction later on in life. If you are getting a craving when hungry, grab a healthy protein snack of nuts and seeds with a medjool date or some dried fruit. Remember we have to eat for energy ONLY, and right, well-balanced nutritional food in our diet can cure a patient better than all the doctors put together. So what you can do today, don't leave until tomorrow, for tomorrow, you may not be here to change!
"Your health is your wealth", and once you have lost it, no amount of money can buy it back. Every organ in your body is a jewel, nurture it.

"Love your body and your body will love you"

Modern packaged foods are always containing some kind of sugar and we have moved away from nature. Going against nature causes the onset of many diseases.

Nature has 5 elements:

1. **Air**
2. **Water**
3. **Sun**
4. **Earth and**
5. **Space**

When oxygen inhalation therapy is used it rejuvenates and detoxifies the organ from stagnant gases.

When water is used it is called hydrotherapy.

When earth is used it becomes a medicine.

When space is used it is called fasting.

I use the principles of cleansing and nourishment, regeneration and rejuvenation of the diseased organ. Toxic substances must be expelled and the body cleansed from inside out before any results can be achieved. It is the buildup of these toxins that cause the issues. Sugar is converted to alcohol before being further broken down by the digestive system and this leaves a toxic residue in the body's tissues.

These poisons which your cells are saturated with, block blood circulation and then the lymphatic system gets blocked and shuts down in various parts of the body and it is the daily buildup of these poisonous toxins that degenerate and deteriorate; triggering off diabetes, liver, pancreas toxicity, arthritis and cancers as the body becomes host to these foreign bodies.

Tune into the power of your mind

The best way to give up addiction of sugar is with the "power of your subconscious mind". When you set your mind to achieve that goal the sky is the limit. You can open your mind to new ideas and introduce healthier foods regardless of age it is never too late. To wait until tomorrow to act is unwise as we never know how long our lives are; tomorrow could be too late.

How consumption of sugar is accelerating the aging process

Toxic foods, combined with excess sugar and salt, fried foods, increased stress levels , and atmospheric pollution, are causing our biological organs to speed up and are increasing the ageing process rapidly. The body gives you several chances to repair, but working against the body's natural healing mechanisms and intoxicating the major organs is resulting in death.

Over time, increased sugar consumption is linked with onset of a variety of health problems, such as heart disease, stomach ulcers (as sugar is acidic), colitis, gall bladder and pancreas diseases, mood swings, overeating and addictive behaviours (such as alcoholism), and disturbed pH levels of skin, blood and urine. Some research shows a link between sugar and alcohol, due to the release of dopamine which is a neuro transmitter in your brain. There is a link between the behaviors of these two addictions which may cause upheaval and dips in blood sugar and moods which activate your pleasure centers.

Here are the different ways modern life styles and food choices are impacting us at different ages:

At 10 plus:

With the kind of food and beverages youngsters are eating, their digestive system is slowing down by 3% every year. Hence children are suffering from being overweight, behavior problems, mental hyperactivity, sleep problems, skin conditions, eczema and dry skin, asthma, hay fever allergies and tooth decay, due to excess sugars in their food.

At 30-40 plus:

The body is less resistant with repeat occurrences of flu's and colds. Low white cell count, which is directly affected by sugar intake, drops by 65%. With excess sugar intake the weakened immune system is making the body less resistant to fight abnormal protein cells which in time bind together to make tumours. Clicking and weakened bones with lowered collagen in the body and disturbed and late sleep patterns cause further degeneration. Over time, I have observed in my clinic how weak the digestive systems are of adults in this age group. Sluggish bowels, bloated ness and flatulence, fatigue, exhaustion and memory loss is also on the increase.

At 45 plus:

With the ingestion of the wrong foods the digestive system is now corrupt. Breathlessness upon little exercise is common and the hardening of the arterial walls of the heart will have started to block the hearts major functions, causing strain.

Free-radical damage to the eyes is on the increase, a condition that once occurred at the age of 70 plus. Erectile problems in men and fertility and menstrual problems in women have doubled with high intake of sweetened fizzy drinks that contain excessive levels of sugar and artificial colourings and sweeteners.

Little exercise and a bad diet, obesity and a couch potato lifestyle, sluggish bowels, and poor blood circulation is a major issue. Muscles do not get their fuel and with the ingesting of amino acids (for toning and elasticity), and water retention has doubled due to lymphatic blockage.

By 60 plus:

The accumulative and degenerative effects of these life style choices are getting worse and worse as we get older. This age is more likely to experience organ failures and complex health issues. Individuals in this age group can pay for regular health insurance policies whilst being uncertain of their health, which has declined so rapidly.

"How fast you age depends on both your physical and mental approach to aging".

There is no doubt that your genetic disposition may play a major role in your health, but eating habits and lifestyle patterns also contribute massively. People are suffering from being overweight, sluggishness, constipation, joint swelling and inflammation, blood pressure issues, cardiac conditions, cataracts on the eyes, memory loss, with tooth decay.

You can overcome and resolve health issues with the guidance of this book when you reflect on and action the recommended changes.

You will have more clarity and be able to tap into your inner self and unwind the maze of imbalances of emotions and habits that you create which start off with a thought, and then an action. This then forms into a habit, and then when that habit is repeated daily without you being fully aware, it becomes second nature. It is not letting you recover and achieve optimal health.

The image of scales on the front cover of my book was my chosen image, indicating a balance of life. Tipping off the scales is when you tip off into an unhealthy lifestyle that becomes a routine to you. Having a well-balanced life will involve taking care of yourself, setting healthy routines, focusing on nurturing yourself, planning your meals, staying positive, reducing stress, socializing and connecting with people outside of work, and staying focused to achieve your goals and aspirations. But don't be disappointed if you have defaulted in achieving a goal. Try and try again!

Each chapter has been created to clearly show the techniques and how to apply them.

I have created a Unique Branded System called Body Balance Blueprint™ utilising what I call the 5 Ss'. These are as follows: Situation, State, Sustenance, Supplements and Sleep. And further more you are given a guide on how to implement the 5 Cs to achieve healing. They are a call for action, and information on how to reflect on your changes leading to recovery.

HERE YOU WILL CELEBRATE!

CHAPTER 1
A LIFE CHANGING MIRACLE STORY

It was a very cold and gloomy morning in the month of February 2018, and whilst I sat writing an article, my phone kept on beeping. As I glanced over at it, I saw that I had received a text message from one of my patients who had become a dear friend of mine. As I was so absorbed in writing my article, I merely glanced at the message, which stated, "Please help me, can you please answer my call, I need help?". At that moment in time I didn't think much of it and I continued to write, but the beeps did not stop. I was receiving one text after another.

"It's very urgent, please help me!".
"Can I please talk to you?"

The number of texts coming in startled me and that's when it clicked that it was a matter of urgency. I immediately replied to say that she should call me and when she did there was a great desperation in her voice to say that she urgently needed help.

"What's wrong, you are calling so early in the morning?",
I asked.

It was so cold and as I peered through the frosted windows I could see snowflakes scattered everywhere. From the tone of her voice I realised that the situation was very serious. Whilst I was speaking to her I could sense a huge cry from the women's heart and soul as she explained that her husband had a serious infection on both of his feet. I asked her how serious it was and whether he was getting treated by the hospital. Again with a great sigh of sadness she said,

"He has deep infection in both his feet and the hospital are considering amputation."

We proceeded in conversation, and I was curious to know why the hospital was considering amputation and why she was letting me know so late in the process. I could hear her crying and so I reassured her that we would get the issue under control.

She said there was no choice, she was not sure whether I could help as they had left it too late. She unfolded the story to me that her husband in December 2017 bought a pair of shoes which were the wrong size. Being a very large man, he decided to buy shoes that were one size bigger than the size that fit him. Being diabetic, he decided by doing so he would be able to slip the shoes on and off more easily without having to bend, thus making it more comfortable for him. But quite naive to the fact that wrong sized shoes were rubbing on sides of the little toes, which resulted in repeated abrasion on the skin. Over the fifteen days, the torn skin rapidly became a life threatening deep skin infection. He wasn't to know that in the long run this had potentially resulted in him having to have an amputation.

I told her that I would make my way to the hospital to see him and to keep her calm. As we walked through the long narrow corridors, which were undergoing construction at the time, we could smell the disinfectant in the air. As we walked in and went over to the bedside, we saw him with both his feet heavily bandaged. This was in a diabetic ward because he was a type 1 diabetic.

I questioned him as to what had happened and he explained about his condition, and that the high readings of his blood sugars was not helping to control the infection and heal the weeping wounds on both of his feet. And to my shock and dismay he also added that he was so lost and confused that he had now signed on the dotted lines and he was waiting for the doctors to give him the report for an amputation surgery.

The infection and abscesses on both of his feet in December 2017 had led to deep tissue infection and further progressed to gangrene. He had lost all feeling in his feet and skin. He had been admitted into hospital in January 2018 with serious grade 4 infection and his feet had been heavily bandaged due to nine pockets of pus and weeping wounds on both feet. His job was in jeopardy due to over two months admission in the hospital. He had taken numerous anti-inflammatory drugs and antibiotics administered intravenously but his infection had not reduced, and both of his feet had been plastered for six months.

Eventually the doctors turned up and I listened to the them say to him that they had now marked him for amputation and they asked him whether he was ready.

He replied "Not really but I have no choice". So I asked the doctors what was happening and whether they could give him a few days to think about it.

The dinner ladies came into the ward with the meals that had been pre-ordered by the patients and I was shocked to see that the meal that he had chosen were all starchy carbohydrates and high in sugar, it had cabbage and potato and he also took a fruit sponge which I explained was a very bad choice considering he was taking insulin for type 1 diabetes as well as the tablets for type 2 diabetes.

He asked "What shall I do?" So I told him that he would

have to leave the hospital for me to assess him and see if I could treat his infected wounds and speed up the healing process. So they made some excuses and got out of the hospital the following afternoon.

When I got to his house at three o'clock, I insisted that they open the bandage. They were reluctant as the bandage was just refreshed and it was highly medicated with anti-bacterial spray.

When his wife opened the two inch thick bandages, I was horrified to see that the infection was so deep and so severe that there were nine pockets of pus below the side of both his little toes, over an inch in length. The area was already dark purple and he had no feeling on his skin and the top arch of both his feet. The infection was quite close to the bone and the only reason for amputation was to stop the rest of the leg from becoming infected. When I saw the infection with the smell of the wound so gross , I began to wonder as to how this infection could be brought under control. Due to the bacteria on the base of his infected skin, I insisted that they not bandage the feet anymore. He could barely walk, and the moment he tried to walk he was seeping blood and fluid from the wound, I advised him that it would have to be left dry, so I instructed him to only bandage lightly and only walk to the washroom.

I went back to my clinic and picked up my LED light treatment as I thought this would be the best form of treatment for him.

Having administered the tri-light therapy in a structured way (red, blue and near infrared light), I noticed within the first 24 hours there was a change in the wound and skin tone.

The tri-light treatment was a life saviour for him as after two and a half days with sixteen treatments, which I administered in the comfort of their home, he was showing amazing recovery. He had no more weeping wounds. He could put weight on his feet without the wounds seeping pus. Miraculously, over the remainder of the days, he had new skin collagen and tissue repair.

He took on my instructions and cancelled his routine hospital and nurse appointments to bandage his wounds. I had insisted on the exposure of the wound, and to use the sprays and the remedies I had prescribed. Whilst I administered the tri-light treatments tirelessly over, ten days he walked back into the hospital without any bandages.

To the shock of the doctors and nurses and their observations, they suggested that he did not need amputation or plastering. Within three weeks he started going to work part-time, and a few weeks later he was able to return to work full time!

Do remember this phrase "a stitch in time saves nine". Never allow these kind of situations to escalate to the point that it is too late, and to the point that it seriously endangers your health and wellbeing. A little effort taken in time to fix a small problem will prevent it from becoming larger and requiring more effort to treat and heal. It is better to deal with problems immediately, as you will be jeopardizing your condition, which may get worse and will certainly take longer to heal.

Through the process of healing, I had to radically change his diet and remove all the hidden sugars and simple carbs. I also helped him to develop a positive mindset and helped him create healthier thoughts that would help him feel confident and which would have a direct impact on his conscious and subconscious mind. This aided him to reach further healing. It is always great to pursue a path of positive healing by keeping your anxiety down, creating calmness within yourself.

In any life situation, if you feel unwell, try to take control of your thoughts and give your body permission to heal. It is with these thoughts that the healing process begins and on a conscious level you speed it up. By doing so all barriers can be broken despite of what your medical reports show and what doctors may suggest.

Remember you are under the direction of your own consciousness and you'll be amazed and surprised at how much you can speed up your own healing process with the feel good factor. It can work miracles in your life and as you see for my patient it was life changing, so much so that he has not had any amputation and is living a healthy life.

CHAPTER 2
THE 5 S'S OF HEALTH

 $\mathbf{H}$ ealth is like having savings in your account and being sick is an expensive choice to make. Being healthier in the short term might appear to be an expensive choice but in years to come it will pay off. This means manifesting smart choices.

In today's Twenty First Century, do you agree that we have to make SMART choices? You may have a smart car or a smart watch. We are living in the world of smart. We are conditioned every day, to buy smart products that give us more options to save time and increase productivity. The media industry is conditioning us but so is the food industry. It's conditioning us every day to want to eat certain foods. The worst food adverts are put on the television at peak times when children are watching, so their minds are conditioned to want those foods. In a world where we are conditioned, we need to take back control and implement our own life rules and regulations that benefit us genuinely, rather than just benefiting the profit margins of large corporations. This is why I have created the Body Balance Blueprint ^{TM} .

The Body Balance Blueprint ^{TM} will help to improve your mind, body and general lifestyle. By making the right choices you become free from pain and you wake up in the morning feeling vibrant, with good positive thoughts about what you want to achieve in your day. You have the tools to then achieve those goals. Imagine going from a state of negativity and getting into the state of positivity and having wellness and a healthier balanced life where your work will not be jeopardized.

I have created my very own Body Balance Blueprint™ that has been created around my Unique Branded System (UBS) as shown below.

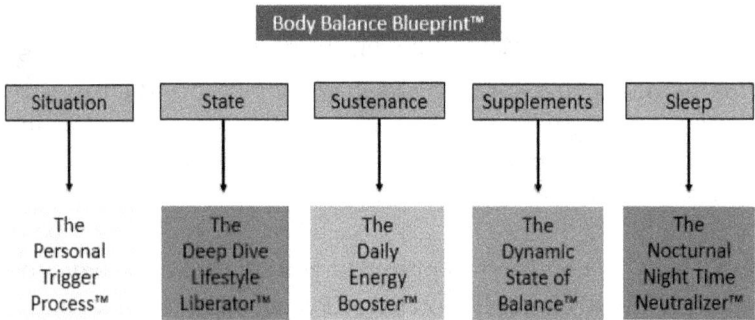

The 5 S's of health are as follows:

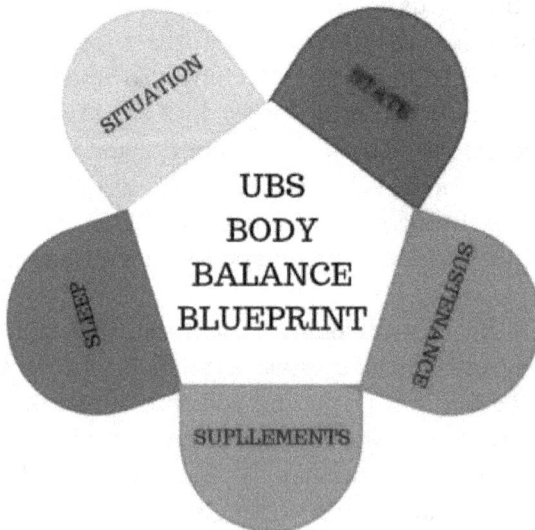

SITUATION

Good health is a cherished gift and its importance is undeniable. A health problem can arise whenever the body is not getting enough nutrition, is lacking the essential vitamins and minerals or is getting too much of them. A balanced diet rich in essential vitamins and minerals is crucial but is often overlooked in daily life. For example you may ignore the daily breakfast habits you have in your family such as eating a lot of fatty foods, and after a while when your body starts bloating and informing you to take immediate notice, only then do you start to take action.

You have to assess the behavior that is causing the situation of ill health. It could be eating the traditional breakfast eaten in your culture that is causing you discomfort.

Steps to uncover the cause of ill health include:

- **Past:** Consequence of repetition of the same foods
- **Explore:** Those things that are probably affecting you, i.e. bloating systems due to wheat, dairy etc.
- **Present:** What you are doing now
- **Evaluate:** The situation
- **Amplify:** one diet does not suit all

The term "situation" stated in the Body Balance Blueprint™ refers to how individuals evaluate what their bad habits are when eating.

Case study:

I had a 50 year old patient who would start their morning with a cup of tea and that was their regular routine. But I had to assist them to break this habit to overcome the bloatedness and heart burn symptoms they were experiencing. Once the patient took responsibility and made the necessary changes, she overcame the symptoms. With support with her food changes, she improved, and the remedies given to her helped heal the lining of her stomach.

"IT IS THE MIND THAT ALTERS THE HABIT."

STATE

It has been proven through various research that certain food has a drastic effect on your mood. For example, chocolate releases stress and gives you the feeling of being in love. Similarly, fast food is packaged and presented to us in a way that is extremely appealing, and this affects our subconscious mind, and in turn we tend to eat more of these foods.

It is often observed that most people overeat the wrong type of food when they are sad and depressed to relieve stress. Similarly with anger, we might eat a food item that we like, which can cause discomfort to our overall health. Overindulgence can have serious risks to overall health and well-being.

There are also other factors controlled by our state of mind, which is the timing of eating food. There is a biological clock in all of us which corresponds to the call of nature. If you divert from the right time of eating and have an irregular sleep pattern, this is going to have adverse effects on your health. The state of your health can also be affected by the blue light syndrome, which occurs due to extensive exposure to laptops, TV's, mobiles or any form of screens at night, or watching violent movies before bedtime.

The optimum time to have breakfast is 7am, the best time for lunch is 12pm and the best for dinner is 7pm depending on the country GMT time zone. Leaving dinners later than 7pm increases the load on the liver which has to break up your food whilst you are asleep. Many people are less active in the evening, so calories are not burned. Research has shown that breakfast is the most important meal of the day.

Our environment, family background, education and life experiences play a very important role in keeping our emotions positive or negative, if your family and friends are cheerful and can boost you up when you are feeling negative, it yields positive results. When you are in a positive mood, you are likely to make positive decisions, whereas, if you are in a negative mood, you are more likely to engage in negative behaviors. Overly optimistic and overly pessimistic attitudes hamper your ability to take a decision without exercising a bias, excessive emotions result in clouded thinking, and these both lead to poor decision making.

Steps to uncover the cause of ill health include:

- **Past:** look at your emotions which are tampering your mind
- **Explore:** a new way of creating harmony
- **Present:** look at your behavior and actions once your mood is effected
- **Evaluate:** acknowledge your thoughts
- **Amplify:** bring humor and light heartedness to your emotions

Case study:

With the state of her mind my patient always made a bad choice of food when she was in stress or under emotional distress. She would rush to have high sugar containing foods, chocolates, packets of boiled sweets and then she would have mood swings. When she understood what was happening with her dips in sugars, she began to take control of her actions and made healthier alternative choices.

"THINK BEFORE YOU ACT."

SUSTENANCE

There is always a choice involved with food and the lifestyle you want to adopt. It is noted that people with a healthier lifestyle also do look at having a healthier choice of food. Healthier diet includes a variety of protein, green vegetables, fruits and other healthy choices. They can make you feel light and fresh and equip your body with all the essential minerals and vitamins and other necessary things needed to keep you healthy and fit.

On the contrary, an unhealthy diet, which includes a range of fast food, excessive carbohydrates, and similar things can result in various ailments and can cause serious health issues. Whenever you are eating something consider the following in your mind: the food that you've eaten; has it made you lazy, sleepy, and tired? From that, you can generate information to find the culprit. That particular food might be an allergy or a sensitivity for you.

Sustenance and diet are essential and most crucial are the nutritional values of what you are eating. We need to ask the questions: what temperature was the food cooked in? What pan was the food cooked in? How was it presented and how did you eat it? Were you sitting, standing or driving, or on the go? If you're in motion and you're feeding yourself, your body does not resonate.

Try not to eat when you are angry or stressed because in that frame of mind you will not chew thoroughly. In this state of mind, your emotions are in turmoil and you gulp your food down too quickly.

It is best to take sensible actions to calm your nerves down, by sitting in a relaxed environment and employing relaxation techniques that work for you.
Chewing and making conscious effort with your teeth as you

masticate each bite is of paramount importance, as it is through the saliva in the mouth that we start the digestive process.

As chewing breaks down your food into smaller particles it will be much easier for the stomach to further break down the food with the digestive enzymes and it will be easier for your small intestine to further absorb the nutrients which have passed down from the stomach.

Whilst you are chewing slowly you will also be able to savor and enjoy all the flavours of the food on your plate. Moreover when large undigested particles enter the intestines you may feel bloated, suffer from flatulence, constipation, irritable bowel symptoms and cramping.

Steps to uncover the cause of ill health include:

- **Past:** look at the repetitions and addictions of the food which are causing you discomfort
- **Explore:** make the right choice of food with the practitioners advice
- **Present: aim** to focus on improving your digestion
- **Evaluate:** avoid foods that are causing you discomfort
- **Amplify:** have a varied diet

Case study:

When you understand the reasons behind your situations and states you will be able to make wiser choices of food. Whatever the situation at the time, you should evaluate and think about how you will burden you digestive system with the wrong choice of food.

A classic case was of a 45 year old patient who had serious candida thrush symptoms and when in stress she would finish a box of chocolates or Indian sweets. Her thoughts caused her to take action to indulge her into making the wrong choices. Her comfort was the triggering factor, and it was her weakness, and it lead to the repeat flare ups of candida thrush which gave her many days of discomfort. But to break away from her repetitive habit, I had to get her to understand that she was victimising her body. Medicine will only work if she took action on the choice of food.

I put her on a one week trial diet that incorporated nuts and seeds as snacks and to her surprise her symptoms of thrush improved dramatically and the Ayurveda remedies I prescribed had a much better impact.

> "DON'T BECOME A VICTIM OF OVER INDULGENCE. ANY OVER EATING OR REPETITIVE FOOD CAN TRIGGER SENSITIVITY'S OR ALLERGIES."

SUPPLEMENTS

Supplements help to balance the level of different essential nutrients in your body. You need to have supplements in your diet because of soil depletion. They must be taken under practitioner's advice. Many people take supplements at their own discretion and they may not know how effective they are and how much they are being absorbed and assimilated as the supplements leave the gut.

You need to consider the source of your supplements and be wary of online products. Most supplements are leaving the colon bound without being broken down. Getting to a practitioner and getting the best advice to see which product best suits, which you can achieve either through a scan or through a physician or a dietitian, will get you the best information.

Sadly in the Twenty First Century, with modern farming techniques, heavy usage of fertilizers, and agricultural sprays and pesticides, there has been a huge reduction in the vitamin and mineral content of the fruits and vegetables we are eating. However, the use and intake of organic fruits and vegetables may give you sufficient nutrients, but it also depends on how we cook our food and at what temperature.

Intake of supplements such as essential fatty acids, vitamins and minerals and phytochemicals with a practitioner's advice, protect, repair and regenerate our cellular structure and organs in the body. Supplements boost your immune system, keeping body and hormones balanced. Supplements can aid in blood sugar balance, blood pressure, cholesterol, and help with oxidative stress which is vital to maintain good health. It can also help with muscle repair, assist in rebalancing your body after surgical procedures, enhance your health and boost your energy. Replenishing nutrients after a workout, recharges your energy levels and helps with a reduction in oxidative stress.

Steps to uncover the cause of ill health include:

- **Past:** try to summarize your past health i.e. injuries, allergies etc.
- **Explore:** your deficiencies in your daily food protocol
- **Present:** list how your energy varies throughout the day
- **Evaluate:** assess how the supplements that you're taking are being absorbed
- **Amplify:** assess whether you are meeting your nutritional goals

Case study:

Heavy usage of pesticides in agriculture and farming to get

better yield in quantity but not quality of food has certainly not been kind to mankind. In addition the way we cook our food on high heat may be destroying the vital vitamins and minerals.

With the heavy usage of pesticides in modern agriculture, which is focused on better yields and not better quality food, we have experienced declines in our health, and hence we need to support our body with vital vitamins and minerals that are essential to catalyze and help our bio chemistry to work. But it must be followed up with doctors or with practitioner's advice. There is too much on the market to confuse you and some cheap supplements do not get absorbed at all and may only give you a placebo effect.

The most shocking case I had was of a couple who bought a cheap brand of Vitamin B and for 20 years consumed the same product every day. Thank god it was a cheap tablet which was probably not absorbing properly and they showed no side effects of long term use of Vitamin B.

"WITH THE RIGHT CHOICE OF THE PRODUCT YOU WILL HAVE A POSITIVE OUTCOME."

SLEEP

Are you waking up feeling fresh, rejuvenated and rested to face the day? Or have you turned off the snooze button several times to get a few minutes extra sleep?

The previous day's activities could affect your sleep as it may result in you having light and broken sleep, a sleep with vivid dreams, or a deep rested sleep. Assessing the cause and implementing a change in your behaviour, thoughts, stress management, and choice of food including the right supplements, will help you to have better quality of sleep.

Sound sleep plays a vital role in your physical health. Sleep can be affected by your thinking, your emotions, poor eating, indigestion, heartburn, feeling bloated when you lie flat, lack of good exercise, illicit recreational drugs and intake of caffeine. All these things can reduce your total sleep time.

The importance of a good night's sleep cannot be stressed enough. Sleep is essential for the body to function correctly. If you are not giving your body the rest it needs, it most certainly will not perform correctly.

Sleep deprivation can lead to various illnesses which can have adverse effects on health.
 Here are a few things to help you understand the importance of sleep and its connection with your overall health and well-being.
Sleep is essential. While you're sleeping the liver is performing over 400 functions.

Try to assess what time you're eating your food. If you've eaten very late and gone straight to bed and not given yourself that three hour gap then throughout the night your liver is going to carry on like a machine.

By not giving yourself a three hour gap, your body has a mammoth task of digesting the food and metabolizing and absorbing the meal . This will disrupt your sleep and the calories in the food will probably be stored as fat and will be detrimental to your metabolic health. However for those who are diabetic, a light snack is advised to keep blood sugars balanced.

Good sleeping postures include sleeping on your back with knee support, or sleeping on your side with a pillow between your knees. Getting into bed between 8pm to 12pm will allow for adequate sleep, including both restorative and dream rich sleep, and the most restorative beneficial sleep is between the hours of 2am to 4am.

It is claimed that the timing people are exposed to blue light from devices should be taken into consideration as it can prevent quality sleep. Short wavelengths affect the levels of melatonin more than any other wavelength does. Normally, the pineal gland in the brain begins to release melatonin a couple of hours before bedtime, and melatonin reaches its peak in the middle of the night.

Steps to uncover the cause of ill health include:

- **Past:** why was your sleeping deprived?
- **Explore:** what actions do you take before you go to bed which result in deprivation in sleep
- **Present:** how rested is your sleep? What kind of sleep are you having i.e. deep state of mind or dream sleep?
- **Evaluate:** how you can improve your state of sleep, i.e. have a calming herbal tea
- **Amplify:** do not take your worries to bed

Case study:

Sleep deprivation is another very common symptom I have to address with my patients, and I help uncover the reasons and causes behind it, and I assist my patients with the right products or my Ayurveda complexes.

My 20 year old patient was suffering from sleep issues due to her childhood bullying. When we worked to uncover her deep pain and fears of rejection, I was able to help her improve her sleep. She found her self-worth and self-love and with guided meditation practices she learnt to switch off her over active mind.

"DO NOT TAKE YOUR WORRIES TO BED, BE GRATEFUL FOR YOUR DAYS EVENTS."

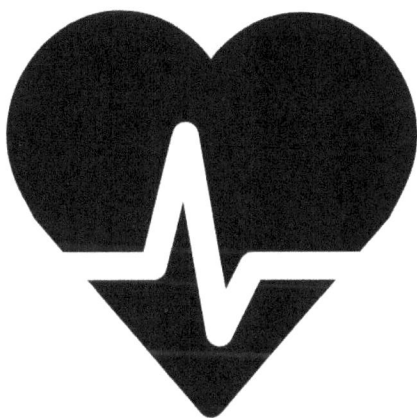

GOOD THOUGHTS ARE LIKE FRAGRANCE & ESSENCE OF ROSES AND BAD THOUGHTS ARE LIKE THE THORNS OF A ROSE STEM.

CHAPTER 3
BRAIN FOOD CONNECTION

There are five types of brain waves, and we can understand how to optimize them for better sleep, mindfulness, productivity and general wellbeing.

Our brain exhibits habitual electromagnetic patterns on a day to day basis, and these are directly linked to our states of mind.

Now what are brain waves? Are they actually a physical thing?

Contrary to what you may think, brain waves are not actually a physical thing; however they are the measurement of activity that is going on within your brain.

If you hooked up enough wires to your scalp you would be able to power a light bulb and that's why the brain is known as an electrochemical organ. The brain is comprised of neurons which are specialised brain cells that transmit information throughout the body in both chemical and electrical forms. The electrical communication wired by these neurons are measured in the form of brain waves.

There are five types of brain waves:
1. Gamma
2. Beta
3. Alpha
4. Theta
5. Delta

Gamma waves are high frequency waves that are connected to insight, peak focus, and expanded consciousness. These waves are generated when we are learning new information, sharply concentrating, or storing memories.

Beta waves allow us to concentrate hard on tasks and they're critical for when we read, write, and socialise. However the downfall of these waves are that they can deteriorate our energy and reduce emotional awareness and creativity.

Our alpha waves are associated with relaxation and reflection. These are the waves that kick in when we've just got home after a long and tiresome day and we want to wind down and relax.

Finally there are the theta waves and delta waves which are associated with sleep. Once you fall asleep you experience the theta waves which are associated with dream sleep, and delta waves corresponds to deep, healing sleep.

All these brainwaves can be manipulated through meditation, and this is referred to savasana in Yoga practices. Regular meditation has been found to increase alpha activity and decrease beta in waking states. It's also been demonstrated to enhance gamma wave states, which makes sense because gamma is thought to increase awareness and make us very in tune with ourselves and our environment.

How is the brain connected with food?

THE BRAIN

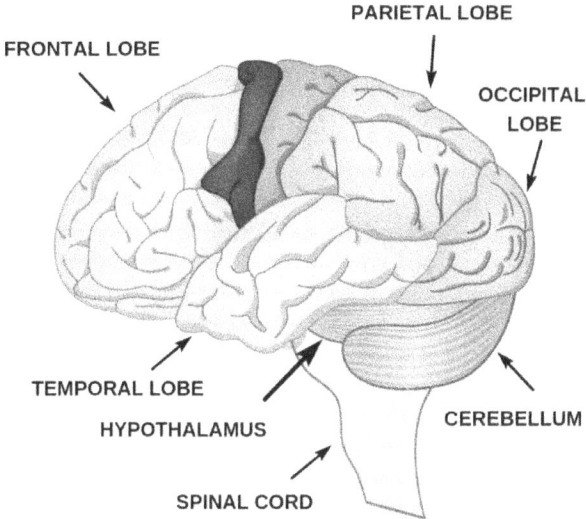

FRONTAL LOBE

PARIETAL LOBE

OCCIPITAL LOBE

TEMPORAL LOBE

HYPOTHALAMUS

CEREBELLUM

SPINAL CORD

HYPOTHALAMUS CONTROLS
APPETITE AND METABOLISM

There is a logical reason why food makes us salivate. Our brains subconsciously react to the smell, sight and even thought of food with the increased secretion of saliva. This is because we need saliva to help our teeth to chew and prepare food to be digested.

Saliva is 99.5 per cent water and 0.5 percent proteins, electrolytes and lipids (a group of natural occurring molecules).

Amylase, a protein enzyme found in saliva, begins the process of breaking down food before it enters the stomach and intestines.

The nerves that control saliva production are part of a reflex system that is activated subconsciously when you are eating. The smells, tastes and even the movement of your jaw muscles can activate this reflex.

The part of the brain responsible for this salivary reflex is the medulla oblongata which controls a variety of functions from sneezing to vomiting. On receiving these stimuli, the medulla oblongata sends neurotransmitters to the glands to produce the saliva.

Now, I am going to go in to detail about what makes us hungry, full or lose our appetite.

Hunger

Hunger is a normal sensation that makes you want to eat. Your body tells your brain that your stomach is empty. This makes your stomach growl and gives you hunger pangs. Hunger makes some people feel lightheaded or grouchy. Everyone is different. Hunger is partly controlled by a part of your brain called the hypothalamus, your blood sugar (glucose) level, how empty your stomach and intestines are, and certain hormone levels in your body.

Fullness

Fullness is a feeling of being satisfied. Your stomach tells your brain that it is full. Normally, this feeling causes you to stop eating and not think about food again for several hours.

Fullness is partly controlled by the hypothalamus, your blood sugar, and having food in your stomach and intestines.

Appetite

Appetite is a desire for food, usually after seeing, smelling, or thinking about food. Even after you feel full, your appetite can make you keep eating. It can also stop you from eating even though you are hungry. This might happen when you are sick or feeling stressed.

Now experts know that hunger is regulated by a complex system of chemicals that send signals between your brain and your body.

The cells in the hypothalamus communicate with cells in other parts of the brain to coordinate the release and uptake of chemicals that help regulate how much and what you eat.

Food triggers the brain to turn the desire to eat into the act of eating. How a food smells, what it looks like, and how you remember it tasting excite chemicals within your brain. The breakdown products of foods such as amino acids from protein, fatty acids from fat, and glucose from carbohydrates, regulate hormones such as insulin, which affect the process at a cellular level. They send messages to the brain telling it that fuel is needed i.e. food.

When the body needs nourishment, neurotransmitters are released. One neurotransmitter called Neuropeptide Y (NPY) is important in sending messages to various parts of the brain. Scientists have recently identified two chemicals, ghrelin and leptin, circulating in the blood that communicate with NPY.

WHAT IS GHRELIN?

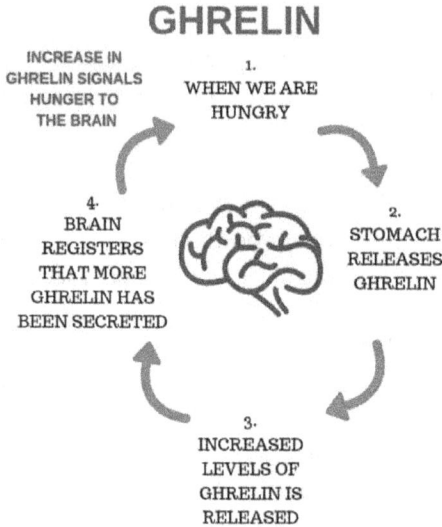

GHRELIN

INCREASE IN
GHRELIN SIGNALS
HUNGER TO
THE BRAIN

1.
WHEN WE ARE
HUNGRY

4.
BRAIN
REGISTERS
THAT MORE
GHRELIN HAS
BEEN SECRETED

2.
STOMACH
RELEASES
GHRELIN

3.
INCREASED
LEVELS OF
GHRELIN IS
RELEASED

Ghrelin is known as the 'Hunger Hormone'. It plays a key role because it signals the brain to eat.

Theoretically, low levels of glycogen and low blood sugar levels stimulate a spike in ghrelin and NPY's activity in the hypothalamus. As NPY is stimulated, your desire for sweet and starchy foods goes up. And when ghrelin rises, so does appetite.

While you sleep, your glycogen and blood sugar stores are used up, causing the brain to release NPY. Skipping breakfast increases NPY levels so that by afternoon, you're set up for a carbohydrate binge. This craving for carbs is not the result of a lack of willpower; it's an innate biological urge at work.

WHAT IS LEPTIN?

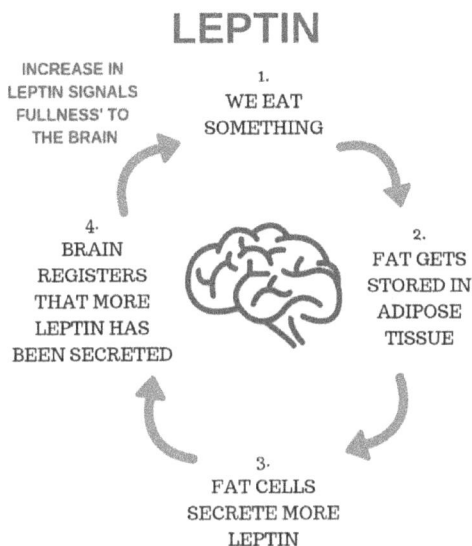

LEPTIN

INCREASE IN
LEPTIN SIGNALS
FULLNESS' TO
THE BRAIN

1.
WE EAT
SOMETHING

4.
BRAIN
REGISTERS
THAT MORE
LEPTIN HAS
BEEN SECRETED

2.
FAT GETS
STORED IN
ADIPOSE
TISSUE

3.
FAT CELLS
SECRETE MORE
LEPTIN

Leptin is a hormone that is released from the fat cells located in the adipose tissues. The hormone sends signals to the hypothalamus in the brain and helps regulate and alter long-term food intake and energy expenditure. The primary role of leptin is to help the body maintain its weight.

After eating, leptin levels increase and inhibit the firing of NPY, so you feel full. If it has been a while since you've eaten, your blood levels of glucose are low and therefore leptin is low, and ghrelin is high.

The circulating levels of ghrelin peak at different times depending on when you have your heaviest meal. People who eat big lunches show ghrelin peaks at a different time than people whose main meal is at night.

To have a healthier lifestyle follow these suggestions:

1. Upon waking, drink two glasses of good mineral water to rehydrate your body. There are great benefits to drinking water on an empty stomach first thing in the morning as it helps to cleanse the colon, flushing out toxins from the body.

As our body is made up of 70% water it helps us to rejuvenate, increases the absorption of nutrients, prevents constipation, and helps with better digestion. Hydration is the most important thing for our body. Water also keeps our lymphatic system flowing and balanced. Hydrating your body also helps us to fight against infections.

A lot of Japanese studies have proven that having water on an empty stomach can get rid of several issues, such as headaches and constipation, as the kidneys cleanse the toxins from the bladder, and the water keeps the stomach pH levels balanced. Water with pH levels of 7.5-9.5. eliminate toxins from the body which leave the skin healthier and looking more hydrated, plump and glowing.

Drinking water at least an hour before food will help to reduce the quantity we eat, but avoid it whilst eating. Often people think they are hungry but most often they are thirsty.

2. Eat a high protein breakfast i.e. have a target of 25g+ of protein preferably gluten free. Do not eat large meals. Finish a meal when you're slightly less than full

3. Reduce the amount of carbohydrates. Limit carbs but don't cut them out completely

4. Never eat after dinner. Finish eating at least three hours before bed

5. Eat three meals a day. Allow 5-6 hours between meals and

if you need to snack, opt for healthy snacks of low glycemic foods such as oat meal crackers with avocado and unsalted popcorn, nuts, seeds or a portion of raw vegetables i.e. carrots, cucumbers, celery sticks, raw courgettes with homemade hummus.

HYDRATE, HYDRATE, HYDRATE!

Keeping hydrated is key to a healthy lifestyle. There are so many benefits in relation to the consumption of water.

The key benefits are listed below:

- Increases brain power and provides energy.
- Promotes healthy weight management and weight loss.
- Flush out toxins.
- Improves your complexion.
- Maintains regularity.
- Boosts immune system.
- Prevents headaches.
- Prevents cramps and sprains.
- Maintains the balance of body fluids.
- Helps regulate body temperature
- Prevents backache
- Prevents bad breath
- Helps to overcome hangovers
- Lifts your mood
- Reduces stress
- Improves fitness
- Increases energy
- Relieves fatigue
- Essential for kidney flushing and other body functions
- Helps to form saliva
- Delivers oxygen throughout the body
- Helps with digestion

- Helps maintain blood pressure
- Boosts performance during exercise
- Helps with urinary tract infection

Know your body type

Everyone can be categorised into three different body types.

The table below details the characteristics of each. Which one do you come under?

You may be one of three listed body types or be a bordering between two of them. If you can assess what body type you are, you can determine what physical activities would be suitable for you and what you should be eating and how your body will respond to digesting the food. You may have an ecto body type. These types can consume high carbs without gaining weight. But for meso and endo body types, if they eat foods high in carbohydrate, it will only burn off if they are more physically active. Otherwise they will gain weight and may find it hard to lose. Hence knowing your body type can make a difference in fine tuning your daily nutrition and training, (following a disciplined plan that will become a routine).

Sometimes easier said than done but with determination and coaching guidance you can achieve your goals. Once you have understood your body type you will be able to understand and leverage your knowledge to achieve optimum results.

ECTOMORPH	MESOMORPH	ENDOMORPH
Typically skinny	Athletic & rectangular shape	Soft and round body
Small frame	Hard body with defined muscles	Typically short and stocky
Lean muscle mass	Naturally strong	Gains muscles easily
Doesn't gain weight easily	Gains muscle easily	Gains fat very easily
Flat chest	Gains fat easier than ectomorphs	Finds it hard to lose fat
Small shoulders	Broad shoulders	Slow metabolism
		Large shoulders

The difference between good and bad bacteria

As a Colon Hydro therapist, I have always promoted the use of good healthy bacteria to support the gut system and digestive tract, but I also highly recommend having a few sessions of colon hydrotherapy (colonics) every year. However, the procedure of colon hydrotherapy is advised after a consultation and may not be suitable for a person suffering from inflammation of the colon or a bowel disease.

There are numerous benefits to having colon hydrotherapy. They prevent bloated ness and constipation; help you achieve better sleep, remove toxins, and increase energy and mental clarity. These will be discussed in more detail in the chapter on therapies.

"Good" bacteria, also known as beneficial bacteria, are defined as any bacteria that are beneficial to the body and enhance health. One of the most well-known types of good bacteria are probiotics. Bacteria in our gut help to protect us by crowding out other harmful bacteria that can cause disease. Other good bacteria have been used in medicine to create antibiotics, and others still are used in food production to make fermented foods such as yoghurts.

"Bad" bacteria are traditionally defined as pathogenic bacteria, which means they may cause infection, make us sick or, in some cases, even kill us! Bad bacteria come from external influences such as food, environmental toxins and even the effects of stress on our bodies. Sometimes a disturbance in the force, or an imbalance in the homeostasis of our bodies, will turn a healthy gut microbe into a colony of very unfriendly bacteria inside our bodies.

When our body is stressed, it creates an environment in which the bacteria that were once good or "dormant," can multiply and wreak havoc in our system. Too many antibiotics, bacteria in food, food that isn't prepared well, excess sugar, stress and lack of sleep are some things that can cause an imbalanced body.

Bacteria live throughout our body, but the ones present in our gut may have the biggest impact on our well-being. They line our entire digestive system. Most live in our intestines and colon. They affect everything from our metabolism to our mood to our immune system.

There are different types of gut bacteria such as:
1. Probiotics, which are microorganisms that are believed to provide health benefits when consumed.
2. Whereas prebiotics are gut bacteria which are typically non-digestible, fiber compounds pass undigested through the upper part of the gastrointestinal tract and stimulate their growth.
3. Symbiotic formulations refer to food ingredients or dietary supplements combining probiotics and prebiotics.

There is some evidence that treatment with some probiotic strains of bacteria may be effective in irritable bowel syndrome and chronic idiopathic constipation.

Bacteria in the digestive tract can contribute to and be affected by disease in various ways. The presence or overabundance of some kinds of bacteria may contribute to inflammatory disorders such as inflammatory bowel disease as well as contributing to disorders such as obesity and colon cancer. Alternatively, in the event of a breakdown of the gut epithelium, the intrusion of gut bacteria into other host compartments can lead to sepsis.

How to improve your gut bacteria?

1. Eat a diverse range of foods
2. Make sure to eat lots of vegetables, fruits, beans and legumes
3. Eat fermented foods
4. Reduce the intake of artificial sweeteners
5. Eat prebiotic foods
6. Eat whole grain foods
7. Have a more plant based diet which will help reduce blood pressure, inflammation, cholesterol levels and oxidative stress
8. Take probiotic supplements

As you can see your diet is a crucial aspect to the good health of your body so make sure to focus on having a well-balanced diet.

Methods of cooking

The methods of cooking also play a key role in maintaining good health.

The healthier options of cooking are:

- steaming,
- grilling,
- baking,
- broiling,
- pan fry,
- sautéing,
- roasting,
- pouching,
- stewing.

Even the oils which you use to prepare your food play a major role. There are oils considered healthy as well as some which are considered as bad. While some oils are considered to give us a health boost, others we should be very cautious of. Make sure to choose oils with low saturated fats.

For example canola oil is considered to reduce the risk of coronary heart disease. Flaxseed oil is also good source of alpha-linoleic acid (ALA), one of three omega-3 fatty acids (olive and canola oils also contain omega-3s). You need dietary omega-3s since your body cannot make them on its own. Omega-3 fatty acids reduce inflammation, and thus may help lower the risk of cancers. Avocado oil is high in monounsaturated fatty acids and can promote healthy cholesterol levels and enhance absorption of some nutrients.

The healthy alternative to cooking oils are most commonly known as cold pressed oils which are known to be cholesterol free, are unrefined, unprocessed and do not contain harmful solvents. On the contrary they contain natural antioxidants that are considered beneficial for the body.

The traditional oils that are used for cooking tend to be extracted from seeds, fruits or vegetables and even nuts, whereas cold pressed oils are extracted from oil seeds which may include sesame seed, sunflower seed, hempseed, pumpkin seed, walnut, flax, borage, canola, coconut or olive without using much or any heat to extract as that may degrade the oil's flavor and nutritional quality. The method involves crushing the seeds or nuts and forcing out the oil through pressure.

Cold pressed oils are rich in vitamin E which results in them having healing and anti-inflammatory properties. They also retain healthy antioxidants, which help combat free radicals that cause cell damage in the body, that are otherwise damaged by being exposed to heat. These oils are also a rich source of oleic acid that help boost your immune system. All these oils when cooked on low heat are excellent oils; however, they lose all the nutrients once exposed to too much heat.

These cold pressed oils shouldn't be exposed to a lot of heat which is the sole reason why they are not extracted through heating techniques. These oils have a lot of unsaturated fats which tend to degrade when exposed to heat.

It is recommended that these oils are not used for deep frying or sautéing, as the unsaturated fats may break down making them unsafe for consumption, resulting in them being unhealthy. This is where the method of cooking is crucial. Oils like sesame oil and olive work best when sprinkled over the cooked food. Ensure you are not heating these oils too much. It is recommended that they are used on top of salads, breads and cooked meats to add flavour and to provide a healthier diet.

*HANDS THAT REACH OUT
AND TOUCH
NEVER STOP REACHING OUT
FOR THE STARS.*

CHAPTER 4
THE EMOTIONAL QUOTIENT OF HEALTH

What is Emotional Intelligence?

Emotional intelligence also known as Emotional Quotient is a crucial skill and involves how we understand and manage our emotions in positive ways which defuse conflict, relieve stress and overcome life's challenges. Simply put, EQ is your ability to control emotions.

How does EQ affect the choice of food?

EQ is majorly characterized by self-awareness and self-management. By controlling your emotions, you can effectively manage what you eat and how much you eat. Your food choices are strongly influenced by your level of EQ. Higher emotional intelligence helps you to make good food choices that can contribute to better health. Specifically, if parents have high Emotional Quotient, they will tend to shape a healthy awareness in their children.

Types of eaters

You might be surprised to know that there are multiple types of eaters. They are differentiated on the basis of eating habits and patterns. Some of the commonly found types include:

1. Emotional eater

The emotional eaters eat more when they are happy, sad or stressed. What and how much they eat is determined by their emotions.

2. Compulsive eater

Those who overeat every now and then are termed as compulsive eaters. Their uncontrollable eating is also termed as binge eating. They frequently eat even when they don't feel hungry.

3. Social eater

As the name indicates, social eaters are those who eat more in social settings. Their food choices are influenced by the people surrounding them.

4. Random eater

Random eaters are those who don't eat regular meals. As the name suggests, they tend to eat randomly whenever they want.

5. Mindful eater

The mindful eaters eat carefully and consciously. They avoid overeating and make healthy food choices.

The advantage of being a vegetarian or vegan

The human digestive tract resembles the grass eating animals' gut, and many of the people consider the vegan diet a better option for enjoying sound health. A vegetarian tends to mean that the individual does not eat meat or fish, but there are different types of vegetarians such as;

- Lacto-ovo-vegetarians avoid the flesh of all animals, both meat and fish
- Pescatarians eat fish but no meat
- Lacto-vegetarians consume dairy products but no eggs
- Ovo-vegetarians consume eggs but no dairy
- Vegans avoid all animal-based foods, including honey

Even though vegetarians don't eat meat it doesn't mean to say that they are lacking in certain nutrients needed for good health. Their diet is more plant-based and therefore they usually tend to be more active in making healthier choices of food.

Some of the significant benefits of being a vegetarian include:
- Low risks of diabetes
- Reduced chances of cardiovascular diseases
- Low risks of cataract development
- Reduce hypertension
- Reduced possibility of stroke
- Less incidence of obesity
- Low cholesterol
- Lower risk of developing cancer
- Lead to a longer life expectancy
- Protects against chronic fatigue

Vegetarian foods contain more fiber which is healthier for the gut and includes a variety of foods, vegetables and whole grains. Vegetarian foods are low in unsaturated fats and are therefore very healthy to eat.

The disadvantages of being a vegetarian or vegan

In addition to the number of perks that you get from a vegan diet, there are a few drawbacks as well. Excluding the meat and all the dairy products from your diet can lead to severe nutritional deficiencies. Some common deficiencies are:

- Protein deficiency
- Iron deficiency
- Calcium deficiency
- Low level of Omega 3 fatty acids
- Reduced content of Vitamin B12
- Vitamin D deficiency
- Vitamin B12 deficiency
- Zinc deficiency

To ensure vegetarians and vegans don't lack in these nutrients they need to ensure that they consume plant-based foods which have a good source of iron, vitamin C, calcium, vitamin D, vitamin B12 and zinc .

Such examples of food are:

Iron rich food such as nori, fortified breakfast cereals, legumes, beans and lentils, dried fruit, figs and broccoli.

Vitamin C rich foods such as citrus fruits or tomatoes, which will help the body absorb the iron.

Foods rich in calcium include milk and yogurt. Those who are avoiding dairy products can get calcium from tofu, fortified soy milk, green leafy vegetables, and dried figs.

Vitamin B12 deficiency is greater in vegans and vegetarians in comparison to people who consume animal-based products. The plant-based form of the vitamin cannot be absorbed by the body. They are recommended to take supplements where needed.

Zinc rich foods are fortified cereals, dried beans, nuts and soy products. Zinc is an essential nutrient that plays a role in cell metabolism and immune function.

Becoming a vegetarian will not guarantee good health or a healthy diet. Anyone is at risk of poor health if they eat unhealthily.

Depending on how the food has been cooked, regular consumption of deep fried food may increase the risk of high blood pressure, cholesterol and obesity which are all risk factors for heart conditions. Needless to say consumption of too many calories, unhealthy snacks, too many refined carbohydrates, whole milk dairy products, and junk food, whether meat-based or not can cause havoc on the health of your body.

The awareness and importance of chewing your food

You might have heard about mindful eating. It is essential that you chew your food properly as many digestive enzymes will be released, and larger food particles will be converted into smaller ones. Hence, chewing food favors your stomach and assists in the digestion of food.

Not chewing your food is a habit ingrained in you from childhood and many people do not learn mindful eating practices, so they eat when they are in a hurry or distracted by their surroundings.

Improper chewing of food can lead to various health problems, many of which are overseen. One of them being a condition known as Gastroesophageal Reflux Disease (GERD). GERD is a condition in which the stomach contents (food or liquid) leak backwards from the stomach into the tube from the mouth to the stomach (oesophagus). This action can irritate the esophagus, causing heartburn and other symptoms. The condition can also damage the lining of the throat and esophagus.

Other problems include improper breakdown of food resulting in your intestines finding it harder to absorb vitamins, minerals and other nutrients from the food particles as they pass through. This causes an increased risk of bacterial overgrowth, as the larger food particles cannot be easily and fully digested by your stomach. Therefore some food will be left partially unprocessed. Undigested food results in an increase in bacteria in the colon, which may cause a variety of symptoms including, gas and bloating, diarrhea or constipation, and abdominal pain and cramping etc.

Other health issues include, weight gain and the risk of food poisoning, as the food does not get enough exposure to saliva which contains the enzyme that destroys pathogens that cause serious illness as well as poor oral health.

What you feed your body with matters. Food is like a fuel to your body. Therefore, it is essential that you keep a check on what you eat. You should try a one week challenge. Keep a journal with you and write down every time you eat something. Note down the time you eat and try to eat mindfully. You should also note down how much you eat in every mood.

ONE WEEK CHALLENGE

In the table below make a note of the food you have eaten, at which times they were consumed, along with your moods during that time frame. After a week look back and analyse.

	Food eaten	Time of day	Mood
Monday			
Breakfast			
Lunch			
Dinner			
Snacks			
Tuesday			
Breakfast			
Lunch			
Dinner			
Snacks			
Wednesday			
Breakfast			
Lunch			
Dinner			
Snacks			
Thursday			
Breakfast			
Lunch			
Dinner			
Snacks			
Friday			
Breakfast			
Lunch			
Dinner			
Snacks			

Compare the week to the weekend and how that varies.

	Food eaten	Time of day	Mood
Saturday			
Breakfast			
Lunch			
Dinner			
Snacks			
Sunday			
Breakfast			
Lunch			
Dinner			
Snacks			

CHAPTER 5
EXERCISE AND BODY
TRANSFORMATION

A healthy body leads to a healthy mind, and that is only possible through exercise. There is no person on earth who would deny that exercising does not make him or her feel better about their body and themselves as a whole. To achieve your goal of body transformation, you need to start exercising. For that purpose we have come up with the most effective steps that you need to take in order to achieve your goal of body transformation.

Sign up and don't fool yourself

The first step in transforming your body is getting in the habit of exercising at least three times a week if not daily. Now, do not get me wrong, you can transform your body by exercising at home but, a gym is better. By getting a gym membership you are more likely to get up and exercise because you have spent your money on it. The gym will have the right equipment and a trainer who will teach you how to use them properly. When you do it the right way, you will achieve body transformation a lot quicker than at home.

A lot of new year resolutions are made to lose weight and people sign up to the gym only to appease themselves but then do not regularly attend which defeats the purpose of joining in the first place.

S.T.P (Stop The Procrastination)

To achieve any goal in life, you need to stop procrastinating. It is a toxic habit which becomes a hurdle you need to overcome to achieve success. You can watch workout videos all day long, but your body is not going to transform until and unless you beat procrastination, and get up and head to the gym. Getting yourself to the gym is the hardest part but once you reach there, nothing can stop you from achieving your goal. A good tip to beat procrastination is by creating a list of five exercises that you like and that you will be excited to perform. This way you will not dread going to the gym and your chances of procrastinating will also be less.

The myth of exercising

There are a lot of myths surrounding exercise. Before you start your journey of body transformation, you need to debunk those myths by educating yourself so you will not make mistakes and waste time and will thus achieve your goals more efficiently. For instance, there is a myth which states that if you don't feel sore then you didn't have a good workout. Even though soreness in your body and the workout intensity are sometimes connected, how tired your muscles feel isn't always a good indicator of a solid sweat session. Feeling sore doesn't necessarily mean that it was a great workout. It just means that a significant amount of stress was applied to the tissue. However you can have a great workout and not be sore the next day.

Brisk walks are good exercise,, needless to say that you should be out of breath at the end of the session.

Proper recovery will help prevent achy muscles. In the first 30 to 45 minutes post-exercise make sure to refuel your body by staying hydrated and by getting enough sleep. All of these things can help boost recovery and minimize soreness of the muscles.

Types of good exercise

There is no specific type of exercise that is good for everyone. You should look for exercises that will help you achieve your goal. For instance, cardio is good for losing weight, increasing your strength in your heart and lungs and improve your endurance during a workout. It also increases bone density, reduces stress, better sleep and reduces relief from anxiety and depression. Cardio exercise also raises the heart rate. But, they are not ideal when you are trying to gain weight or muscle.

Increase your happy hormones

Exercising has been known to increase our happy hormones which help in transforming our body as well. You will achieve a lot more when you are happy and when you love your body. You cannot transform it in a healthy way by hating it. To increase your happy hormones, workout in the mornings when the sun is shining. It is also recommended that you indulge in meditation and power yoga to increase your happy hormones.

Flexibility and mobility

Both flexibility and mobility play important roles in the fitness of our bodies. Most people mistake those terms to mean the same thing, yet it is quite the contrary. They do however complement one another.

- ☑ Flexibility relates more to the length of a muscle (bending easily without breaking)
- ☑ Mobility is how a joint moves, its range of motion (the ability to move freely and easily)

Exercising makes your body flexible as time goes by, so be patient. It will happen naturally; you will not even notice how flexible and mobile you have become over time.

The benefits of stretching improves and strengthens your muscles. When you are stretching you will have improved circulation and blood flow. It also enhances joint health, prevents backache and provides relief from muscle cramps.

Flexibility and mobility are both very different in how they can affect your body's workout performance and recovery. As we get older we often tend to lose both flexibility and mobility, so it's important to incorporate both into your regular workout routine.

Ensure to use mobility-based exercises as your warm-up and flexibility based exercises after your workout as part of the cool-down, you'll see better results that should have you feeling stronger, less achy and more confident in how your body moves.

Keep yourself motivated

It is hard to remain motivated and people are more likely to get a bit lazy when they either start seeing results or fail to see any results at all. The best way to keep yourself motivated is by surrounding yourself with things, people, and content that inspires you. By removing those barriers on cold winter days and going with a companion or a friend will also help you feel encouraged and motivated. To achieve your goals track your progress and reward yourself but don't set yourself over ambitious goals, as this may demotivate and discourage you.

Watch body transformation videos, read inspiring success stories or make a pinterest board of your body goals and look at it daily to remain motivated.

In the end, always remember to set up short term and long term goals for yourself as they will be your biggest motivation. Love your body and reward yourself for achieving things you never thought you could achieve. Self-love, no comparison with others and a grateful mindset is what keeps you motivated and accelerates your journey towards body transformation.

*HOLDING A BUNCH OF
FLOWERS, GIVES JOY AND SO
WILL THOUGHTS THAT YOU
GRASP.*

CHAPTER 6
THE PERSONAL TRIGGER
PROCESS™

These are the factors which are related to your emotions and your mind. How do you react to situations of stress? If somebody bugs you how do you respond? What are your emotions? How would you react to negativity? Would you carry that burden throughout the day? Would you feel angry with that person? All these emotions affect our joints and all the emotions affect the gut. Your whole digestive tract, from your mouth to your anal passage covers a huge area, and is 31 feet long, with your gut and your colon being 60 inches long, and your small intestine 23 inches long. So the food you eat has to be good quality, eaten and chosen correctly and your state of mind needs to be correct whilst eating.

Manifesting good choices is core. We always need to analyse the way we sit, stand and our body language.

One of the many wonders of your brain is how masterfully it rationalizes your behavior.

Something occurs, you react, and then your brain instantly concocts a reason for your reaction that seems to justify your behavior even if the reason makes no sense. For example, you get very angry because you can't find a report you were working on. You blame the company for giving you insufficient space, the cleaners for moving things around on your desk, or your boss for giving you a stupid task or deadline. You ignore the reasons you are tired and your patience is thin. You suppress your unhappiness with your boss or your life.

The act of rationalizing is so quick, the best you can do is to recognize when it occurs and choose to consider what else could be causing your reaction. There are five steps which you can take to help you with this issue:

Step 1: Accept responsibility for your reactions.

Accept yourself as powerful individual instead of as a victim to remove the veil of self-deception. When you seek to identify what is triggering how you feel in the moment, you give yourself the chance to feel differently if you want to. You will also have more clarity on what you need to do or what you need to ask for to change your circumstances.

What would your life look like if you were in control of your reactions? How free would you feel if you lived your life by choice? If these questions inspire you to diligently practice the steps for emotional freedom, read on.

Step 2: is to recognize that you are having an emotional reaction as soon as it begins to appear in your body.

Don't judge or fear your emotions. No matter what you learned about the evils of emotions, if you don't recognize your feelings, you can't change them, and this negatively impacts your relationships, job performance, and overall happiness.

If the emotion is related to fear, anger, or sadness, the third step is to determine what triggered the emotion.

What do you think you lost or what did you not get that you expected or desired to have?

Step 3: The strengths that have helped you in life are also your greatest emotional triggers

When your brain perceives that someone has taken something you need away from you, or has plans to take it away, and when you feel like someone is not honoring you, your emotions are triggered.

The quicker you notice an emotion is triggered, the sooner you can discover if the threat is real or not.

Needs are not bad. You have these needs because at some point in your life, the need served you. For example, your experiences may have taught you that success in life depends on maintaining control, establishing a safe environment, and having people around you who appreciate your intelligence. However, the more you are attached to having control, safety and being seen as smart, the more your brain will be on the lookout for circumstances that deny you your needs. The unmet need or threat becomes an emotional trigger.

Step 4: Choose what you want to feel and what you want to do.

With practice, the reaction to your emotional triggers could subside, but they may never go away. The best you can do is to quickly identify when an emotion is triggered and then choose what to say or do next.

Ask yourself, are you really losing this need or not? Is the person actively denying your need or are you taking the situation too personally? If it's true that someone is ignoring your need or blocking you from achieving it, can you either ask for what you need or, if it doesn't really matter, can you let the need go for now?

Choose to ask for what you need, or let it go if you honestly feel that asking for what you need will have no value, or do something else to get your need met.

Step 5: Actively shift your emotional state.

You can practice this step at any time, even when you first notice a reaction to help you think through your triggers and responses. When you determine what you want to do next, shift into the emotion that will help you get the best results.

Relax – breathe and release the tension in your body.

Detach – clear your mind of all thoughts.

Center – drop your awareness to the center of your body just below your navel.

Focus – choose one keyword that represents how you want to feel in this moment. Breathe in the word and allow yourself to feel the shift.

Stop trying to manage your emotions. Instead, choose to feel something different when an emotion arises. This is how you gain emotional freedom.

Environmental surroundings

Your home is your comfort zone which is very important to maintain how you feel for your personal growth and well-being and your environment affects your self-image and sense of self-worth. When children are in a good environment they will feel loved and accepted by their family and parents. In that trusted environment they are likely to have more confidence and a healthy self-esteem. It is noted in modern times, a harmonious domestic environment is a key factor to raising children with confidence who are less likely to have behavioural problems or end up in the wrong company that may take them to smoking and substance abuse. If we don't handle stress and turmoil in that environment, it will demotivate a person and seriously interfere with their family life, future educational experiences and their careers.

All these social factors determine how you react in given situations, factors that may have accumulated over time, based on your domestic and work environment.

HEALTH IS PHYSICAL STATE OF PATIENT,
HARMONY IS MENTAL STATE OF THE MIND OF THE PATIENT,
PEACE IS THE SPIRITUAL STATE AND HEALTHY BODY,
HARMONIOUS, PEACEFUL MIND IS HE DEFINITION OF PERFECT HUMAN BEING.

CHAPTER 7
THE DEEP DIVE LIFESTYLE
LIBERATOR™

W e, as human beings, may develop a hard exterior to show ourselves as strong people but on the inside we are all vulnerable. We focus on things that would please other people, and we step away from tending to our own needs and desires. We could be battling with an injury or suffering from excess mental stress, and no one would come running to us. Since when is stress or depression any less significant than having a wound or broken bone? Doctors dress up a physical injury but no one seems to be as bothered with our mental state, just because it is not visible. We strive for a deep dive lifestyle liberator that would allow us to set ourselves free.

Resorting to the deep dive lifestyle liberator is one emotional factor that will stir up the invisible diseases of the mind. The disease will start with its manifestation when our minds reach its maximum program mode. We tend to not have as much control over what we think as we would like, and we end up consuming a plethora of negative thoughts from our environments and the wider society.

As human beings, we resort to chemical based methods to get better instead of experimenting with natural ways to help.. For instance, we are inclined to take a painkiller to alleviate the symptoms of migraine, but one can also reduce the chronic pain by simply tapping and massaging the back of their necks.

Similarly, practicing meditation is one way to ensure our peace of mind. One is simply required to drink a glass of cool water and meditate for five minutes to release stress from their systems as well as get closer to the nature. When practicing meditation one is required to follow the given pattern:

Focus

Meditation is a proven way to liberate you from all the stress and worries in your world. However, you are required to determine the state of your mind to focus better on the meditating process. When you sit down to meditate, you are required to envisage what the future holds for you. You are supposed to question your beliefs and values to create a better picture for yourself.

A person's long lasting beliefs shape their values, and they will make their choices around these ideas, and this will determine the quality of their lives. A person will be committed to their beliefs as it becomes a part of their nature and it shapes their behavior, their decision making and the actions they take that will impact their life.

Being rigid in your thoughts and actions affect your future decisions, which are central to your social life, career, health and well-being.

Also, you should be able to specify the mental values of your life to focus better on relaxing. The more you are aware of the mental values, the more you focus during a meditation session.

Dealing with stress puts a strain on our minds, which causes us to act and behave differently. Of course, one cannot expect a pleasant response from you while you are trying to cope with stress. Our mind behaves erratically and it stirs up the chemical imbalance in our heads, which deepens the stress that we are trying to cope with.

Once we are past that stage we can focus on meditating easily. We can manifest a mindset that allows us to strive for peace and better things in our lives.

Physiological state

Coping with stress is not only detrimental to our psychological health but, it also transforms our entire psychological state. We tend to develop a unique breathing mechanism and posture under stress. Our body molds itself into an L-posture and we start walking with a hunchback posture.

Our mindset and willpower tends to plummet under stress, and we start manifesting negative thoughts. We cannot think straight, and we often find ourselves binging on comfort food, which is never a healthy option for our bodies. We want to eat anything and everything that is junk food, and we want to steer clear of healthy foods when dealing with stress.

Language

When a person is under immense stress, they tend to use negative and disheartening language. Their selection of words is devoid of any pleasure and the tonality of their voice under stress tends to crack. Stress tends to do things to us that we do not fully realize, and couldn't imagine.

Our statements tend to reflect the beliefs and values of our past, and all we want to do is to liberate ourselves from the pattern of a stressful lifestyle. We tend to question our existence and we tend to question what is wrong and what is right for us.

Of course, you are then required to determine what kind of form you will use to reconnect to your higher self. Meditation allows you to reconnect with life and it allows you to recharge your soul. It allows you to think freely and it motivates you to break the patterns of stress, tension, and everything that has been holding us back.

Diagram to show how stress affects our bodily functions

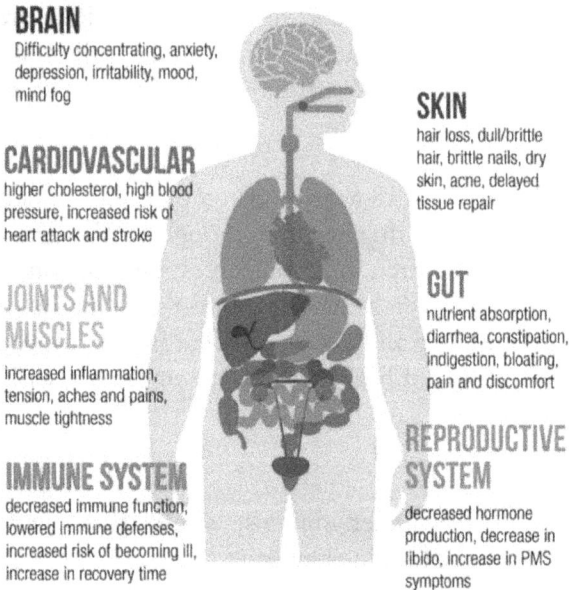

BRAIN
Difficulty concentrating, anxiety, depression, irritability, mood, mind fog

SKIN
hair loss, dull/brittle hair, brittle nails, dry skin, acne, delayed tissue repair

CARDIOVASCULAR
higher cholesterol, high blood pressure, increased risk of heart attack and stroke

JOINTS AND MUSCLES
increased inflammation, tension, aches and pains, muscle tightness

GUT
nutrient absorption, diarrhea, constipation, indigestion, bloating, pain and discomfort

IMMUNE SYSTEM
decreased immune function, lowered immune defenses, increased risk of becoming ill, increase in recovery time

REPRODUCTIVE SYSTEM
decreased hormone production, decrease in libido, increase in PMS symptoms

(Diagram taken from adverse childhood experiences)

CHAPTER 8

THE DAILY ENERGY BOOSTER™

As human beings, we have intrusive and meddling instincts. We have stepped away from the idea of taking care of our bodies and nurturing our souls, and we have integrated unhelpful patterns into our daily lives. We indulge in unhealthy diets, and then, we tend to question our unhealthy diet patterns.

We have become a grazing society, grazing on food all day long. We are urged to resort to a healthier lifestyle but, we have gravitated towards unhealthy junk food. The food industry has introduced tactics and commercials, which are solely dedicated to shape the mindset of the public. They think that posting images of loaded fries and double-decker burgers across the city and social media channels is doing favors for the people. People rush into their nearest fast food restaurant and buy a meal to satisfy their desires.

The packaging of food plays a vital role in playing with the mindset of the people. The processed and harmful foods are wrapped in beautiful packaging and people cannot help themselves but cave in to buying such foods. The packaging of food is changed throughout the year to celebrate various occasions, and people cannot help but cave in to buying bulk foods into their homes. The presence of unhealthy preservatives in foods is detrimental to our health, and it lowers our energy levels significantly. We should start eating energising foods and healthy meals to nurture our body, the way it should be nurtured:

Essential fats - what are they doing for us and the importance of them

Essential fatty acid or EFA's are the types of fatty acids that are usually ingested by humans. It is beneficial for their health. The EFAs are responsible for improving the absorption rate of minerals and vitamins in our bodies. It is also responsible for nourishing our skin, hair, and nails. EFAs are also responsible for improving the functioning of the nerves in our body, and they also help with the production of hormones to ensure normal development and growth.
In addition, the presence of EFAs in our meals is one way to prevent and treat a multitude of diseases.

Stomach pH levels – acid vs alkaline

The pH levels of our stomach tend to vary on some days it would be showing acidic properties, whereas on other days, it would be showing alkaline characteristics. When the pH levels in your stomach becomes acidic it tends to cause inflammation and it makes it difficult for the digestive system to digest food instantly.

On the contrary, if the levels of alkaline are high in your body it makes your stomach susceptible to having gastrointestinal problems.

The importance of raw food in our diet?

We tend to eat a combination of foods on a regular basis; however, we mostly prefer baked, cooked, roasted, fried, or non-raw foods. However, the majority of nutritionists recommend everyone to have a portion of raw food or snack on raw food at least once a day. That portion of raw food will be more nutritious than cooked food and contain more nutrients. You can have a combination of cooked vegetarian or non-vegetarian options and raw greens and vegetables in your meal. Research has shown that raw food nourishes your body in several ways and it supplies vitamins and minerals to your body effectively. You will be getting nutrients from foods that have not been tampered with, and it is the crucial option for you if you have been diagnosed with an autoimmune disease.

What does missing a good healthy breakfast do to you?

It has been forecast that nearly 70% of workers tend to miss their breakfast. Also, two out of four children go to their schools without having eaten anything beforehand.

While skipping breakfast may buy you time to get ready and reach the office on time it is never a healthy option for your body. You will start feeling weak throughout the day, and it lowers your sugar levels significantly. Also, when you try to eat something to cope with the drowsiness or starvation then it would instantly spike your blood sugar which is never a good thing for anyone's body.

Why timing of food is important i.e. not to have late breakfast

A majority of us tend to neglect the timing of eating meals. We tend to eat breakfast late and we also tend to eat lunch and dinner at odd timings. It disturbs our meal intake, and it causes us to eat excessively, which is never a good thing when practicing a diet plan.

One should always eat their breakfast on time, and they should have their dinner at least 3-4 hours before going to bed. If you eat your dinner before going to bed, the meals wouldn't digest instantly and it would cause bloating in your stomach.

Should we snack in between our meals?
The benefits of snacking.

If you are following a diet or if you have a hectic routine, you should definitely eat snacks in between your meals. It re-energises your energy levels and it braces you to perform another task coming your way. The benefits of eating snacks are endless; we have listed a few of the benefits here for you:

- It helps you to feel active and energized throughout the day
- It keeps you satiated if you have a high metabolism
- It improves your cognitive function
- It helps you by improving your focus and concentration
- It helps you to boost your mental health by boosting your physical health

Grab and go – How stress effects our grab and go foods (quick snack foods)

If you have a hectic life, and you are not too keen on having a proper breakfast then, turning to grab-and-go foods is your only option. If you are getting late for work or, you are too busy revising for your test then, you are more likely to grab a snack on your way. However, if you are under stress and you don't want to get stuck in traffic, indulging in quick snack foods become your only option.

If you are grabbing foods on the go there is a high chance that you will binge on the wrong foods, and it would disturb your eating pattern. You could start to skip on healthy breakfasts, and binging on a quick snack would satiate your appetite instantly. It would provide you with fewer nutrients throughout the day, and it could compromise your eating habits and health in the long run.

The benefits of Whole Grain foods (i.e. seeded bread) compared to processed flour foods

When shopping for particular types of foods we need to make the correct informed choices that will benefit our body's whole grain foods are organic and less processed in comparison to their counterparts, and it often requires less preparation time which preserves its nutritional wholesomeness in one way or another.

On the contrary, the processed flour foods contain an unnecessary percentage of carbohydrates in them, which are not usually considered good for your body. Seeded bread contains the right amount of carbs and other nutrients to keep your body's functions steady and normal.

Individuals with allergies to wholegrains and wheat need to make alternative choices.

The benefits of organic vs. inorganic foods

The trend of organic foods has grown immensely over the years, and the majority of health conscious people tend to munch on organic foods in comparison to the inorganic foods. It is not processed or tampered with in any way, and it supplies a wide range of nutrients to our body. It improves the functions of our organs and it helps us to stay fit. On the contrary, inorganic food is processed and fermented, and it is not as nutritious in comparison to the organic foods.

Also, a majority of the farmers tend to use a multitude of sprays and pesticides to keep insects and rodents from preying on the foods; however, it is doing more damage to them than good. Such chemicals are responsible for the depletion of the minerals and other nutrients in the edibles. If you are sensitive to such chemicals then, it would certainly affect your health. Therefore, you should resort to eating organic and naturally grown and processed foods to avoid any sort of health problems.

Food combining

To maintain proper health and have good digestion, food combining must be considered paramount. Improper combinations of food affect your health and creates a load on your digestion. Furthermore it can increase the toxin levels in your body and trigger off digestive disorder diseases. The rules of food combining, if not followed, will make you feel sluggish, bloated, fatigued or sleepy. Often people will not feel appropriately energized or refreshed if the food is heavy with stodgy carbs and the food creates a load on the liver.

With guidelines on food combining you will have improved digestion and will create less strain on the body. You will be able to have better digestion and absorb the nutrients of the food and assimilate properly. You will also be able to have absorbed the necessary micronutrients with a good food combination. Bad food combinations can be a heavy load on the stomach, liver, and the intestine and often noted that people suffer from abdominal pains, stomach cramps, bloatedness, bulging and fluctuance.

When proteins and carbs are eaten in the same meal, the stomach has to release both acid and alkaline solutions which can impair digestion because several types of digestive enzymes need to be released and foods that need to be digested in a short time may take double the time. When this digestion process is slowed down food will putrefy and ferment in your digestive tract resulting in poor digestion and often these undigested food particles can cause food sensitivities and unfriendly bacteria with yeast allergies.

Sit back and think about the daily foods that you are eating from morning until evening.

<u>7 day chart :</u>
Write in the book what you are eating throughout the week.

	BREAKFAST	LUNCH	DINNER
MONDAY			
TUESDAY			
WEDNESDAY			
THURSDAY			
FRIDAY			
SATURDAY			
SUNDAY			

From this week's assessment you can evaluate where you are going wrong.

Table of some examples of good and bad snacks

GOOD	BAD
Mixed nuts	Fried nuts
Mixed seeds	Fizzy drinks
Unsalted popcorn	Caffeinated drinks
Goji berries	Pastries
Dried fruits i.e. dates	Cookies
80% dark chocolate	Donuts
Soya beans	French fries
Avocado	Potato chips
Greek fat free yoghurt	White bread
Hummus with raw vegetables	Deep fried food
Low fat cheese	Candy bars
Whole meal crackers	Processed meat
Hard boiled eggs	Processed cheese
Coconut chip slices	MSG white flour foods
Granola seeded bread	Crackers
Savoury Oat Biscuits	biscuits
Olives	

CHAPTER 9
THE DYNAMIC STATE OF BALANCE™

To remain in a balanced state in our thoughts and behaviors in an ever changing environment is referred to as the dynamic state of balance.

Supplements

Commercial agriculture cultivates food in soil that is depleted of vital minerals. The transportation and logistics of shipping food across long distances and different continents depletes it's freshness and goodness even more Vitamins, minerals, essential fatty acids, super greens, and phytochemicals support the body internally on a cellular and molecular level. In addition, supplements repair and protect our muscular and skeletal system. The high temperature we cook at and the mental state we eat food in will also be a key factor in absorbing the goodness of our food, as stress and eating on the go does not help with absorption. Over a period of years as we repeat such habits, deficiencies may show up in our wellbeing, which is why we may need to substitute them with additional supplementation. Some medical drugs may deplete one or many essential nutrients so supplementing after finding out which one we are deficient in after a blood test is beneficial.

Mind

How is your choice of food affected by your mindset?

Knowing what foods we should and shouldn't be eating can be really confusing, especially when it feels like the advice changes regularly. However, evidence suggests that as well as affecting our physical health, what we eat may also affect the way we feel. If your blood sugar drops you might feel tired, irritable and depressed. Eating regularly and choosing foods that release energy slowly will help to keep your sugar levels steady. If you don't drink enough fluid, you may find it difficult to concentrate or think clearly. You might also start to feel constipated.

How will your emotions be affected by food?

You know that if you eat a sweet snack, such as a candy bar or a sugary donut, you'll get a spike of energy, soon followed by a crashing low. Sugar highs and lows are just one of the many ways food can affect how you feel. Eating a meal will reliably alter mood and emotional predisposition, typically reducing arousal and irritability, and increasing calmness and positive affect. When we are sad, anxious, stressed, angry, bored, happy, we may try to respond to these emotions by eating "comfort" foods. We often use our eating habits to exert control in situations where we don't have control.

Modes of Consciousness

There are two basic modes of consciousness that need to be in balance to allow for the felt experience of wholeness.
Each mode of consciousness reflects particular attitudes that affect how we perceive and shape the way we relate to ourselves, others and situations.

Wholeness is a dynamic state of balance, equanimity and

poise that allows you to move with ease from one mode of consciousness to another, in response to changing internal or external conditions. To make a good decision, a choice that has your best interests and highest good, in mind, you need to be able to shift from one mode of consciousness to another, at will. Creating sustainable lifestyle change does not happen overnight although it always starts with an intention; a choice followed by deliberate action.

How does your left and right brain relate to the food we eat?

The left side of the brain is associated with reasoning, analytic and linear thoughts, numbers, and details. Left brain thinkers rely more on science in food selection and think of calorie counting, nutrients, weight and volume of food, and nutritional theories when making food choices. The right side of the brain is associated with intuition, creativity, and synthesis of parts, feelings, forms, and holistic thoughts. Right brain thinkers rely more on senses in food selection and focus on tastes, colors, aromas, and textures of food as well as how food makes them feel when making food choices.

Body

Dynamic state of body constituents

The concept of a dynamic state of body is defined as how the proteins, nucleic acids, and other components within the cell, are in a continual state of degradation and synthesis. The flow of metabolites through a metabolic pathway at a definite rate and in a definite direction is called the dynamic state of body constituents.

Dynamic state of metabolism

All living organisms, be it a simple bacterial cell, a protozoan, a plant or an animal, contain thousands of organic compounds. These compounds or biomolecules are present in certain concentrations. All the biomolecules have a turn over. This means that they are constantly being changed into some other biomolecules. This breaking and making is through chemical reactions constantly occurring in living organisms. Together all these chemical reactions are called metabolism.

Each of the metabolic reactions results in the transformation of biomolecules. A few examples for such metabolic transformations are removal of CO_2 from amino acids, making an amino acid into an amine, removal of amino group into a nucleotide base, hydrolysis of a glycosidic bond in a disaccharide, etc. We can list tens of thousands of such examples.

How does the mind body connection affect our emotional connection to food?

People who have good emotional health are aware of their thoughts, feelings, and behaviors. They have learned healthy ways to cope with the stress and problems that are a normal part of life. They feel good about themselves and have healthy relationships. However, many things that happen in your life can disrupt your emotional health. These can lead to strong feelings of sadness, stress, or anxiety. Even good or wanted changes can be as stressful as unwanted changes.

Environment

Are we disconnected from mother nature?

With evolution and development humans are getting detached from Mother Nature. Most of us don't even know how it feels to be in the lap of Mother Nature. I've experienced it on mountains, near oceans and in forests. If you'll get out from our concrete jungle then you'll know that you can feel happier there. You forget about yourself when you're in nature. Times slows down there and gives us a very pleasurable feeling. We are abusing and misusing this gift to us left, right and center. The lakes are polluted, the earth is poisoned and the atmosphere is full of toxins, in the name of industrialization.

How lack of sun or sitting in office environments can affect our choice of food

The environment can influence peoples' behaviour and motivation to act. The environment can influence mood. For example, the results of several research studies reveal that rooms with bright light, both natural and artificial, can improve health outcomes such as depression, agitation, and sleep. The places you eat, the way you choose the foods you put on your plate, the people you surround yourself with, where you buy your food, and how that food is presented to you by the culture you live in, all have a serious impact on your decisions.

The importance of supplementation

Vitamins are organic compounds that our bodies use, in very small amounts, for a variety of metabolic processes. It is best to get vitamins and minerals from eating a variety of healthy unprocessed foods. Your body only needs a small amount of vitamins and minerals every day. A varied diet generally provides enough of each vitamin and mineral. However, some people may need supplements to correct deficiencies of particular vitamins or minerals. In the Twenty First Century with the modern farming industry, that use agricultural pesticides and sprays on crops, we do need to have some dietary supplements, on a practitioners advice of vitamins, minerals, herbs, enzymes, amino acids in capsule, liquid or powder form to support the compromised goodness in inorganic crops.

It is commonly believed that taking mega-doses of certain vitamins will act like medicine to cure or prevent certain ailments. For instance, vitamin C is suggested as a cure for the common cold, and vitamin E is widely promoted as a beneficial antioxidant to help prevent heart disease. Supplements make it much easier to get the necessary nutrients to build muscle and can even give you an advantage and enhance your training when taken right and combined with a good diet.

However, you should always consult a qualified health professional first to avoid any drug-nutrient interactions. And avoid supplements with sweeteners, colours, artificial flavours, preservatives, or fillers.

CHAPTER 10

THE NOCTURNAL NIGHT TIME NEUTRALISER™

How sleep is related to health and wellness

The human body has very complex machinery, and constant work can make you feel tired and exhausted. In order to maintain the functional efficiency of the body and to enjoy proper health, sufficient sleep is essential. Lack of sleep can cause multiple health disorders.

Sleep requirements vary from person to person. It depends on different factors including your age, daily routine and lifestyle. The quality of your sleep, and not just the amount of hours you sleep is essential. On average, an adult individual should have 7 to 8 hours of deep sleep per night.

The different kinds of sleep

Basically, there are five different stages of sleep which are divided into two categories including the Non-REM and REM sleep. The first four stages fall under the Non-REM sleep. Each of the sleep phases has a particular purpose. Both the Non-REM and REM phases serve to have a regenerative impact on multiple processes in the body. Besides, our body needs both the deep and light sleep for improving mental capacity.

Is dreaming beneficial and how does it affect our diet?

Dreaming is a healthy activity that can enhance your problem-solving capabilities and improve your creativity. Your dreams also reflect your mindset and these are based on your values and beliefs.

The negative impact of lack of sleep

Lack of sleep can increase your appetite, and you may want to eat more junk food. It is often observed that those who are sleep deprived often crave sugary and junk food which can lead to several digestive issues. Lack of sleep also significantly affects your performance throughout the day. If you fail to enjoy a sound sleep at night, you will wake up tired and fatigued.

Moreover, insufficient sleep can also cause stress and irritability. Simply put, sleep deprivation can negatively affect our body and mind. It increases the chances of diabetes type 2 and contributes to weight gain.

Some people take sleep-inducing pills, but that is not a recommended solution if you are not experiencing chronic insomnia. Taking sleep drugs without prescription can be really dangerous and can cause several side effects including drowsiness, loose stools, and dryness of the mouth.

Couch potato sleep vs cat naps

If you are in the habit of taking short sleep breaks where your mind doesn't switch off completely, you must know that this is not healthy for your body. Straining the posture of your body, and not allowing your mind to rest properly can be really damaging to your physical and mental health. Instead of taking little sleep breaks every now and then, you should take cat naps in the day to cover sleep deficiency. These can be helpful to reset your system and make you feel active and energised.

How to enjoy good quality sleep?

1) Create a routine for your bedtime.
2) Dim the lights in your bedroom, this will help you to unwind
3) Follow a regular sleep schedule
4) Have early supper as heavy meals may make you feel unrested. Avoid snacking before bed
5) Late night gym workouts may delay your sleep as your body releases adrenaline.
6) Avoid caffeinated drinks late in day, as caffeine may put you in alert mode
7) Do not allow yourself to stay in a state of overdrive and overthinking about your day
8.Having soft gentle music with Meditation may be helpful
9)Having a comfortable bed with a suitable mattress, pillow and duvet is equally important
10) Using a hot water bottle may assist you in drifting off to sleep quicker

Connecting with mother nature

Instead of taking pills for sleep, you should look for some natural remedies. For instance, you can include some physical activity such as exercise or taking a walk in your daily routine to enjoy good quality sleep.

Selection of sleep environment

If you want to enjoy a sound sleep, it is essential to choose the environment carefully. Trying to sleep in a noisy place can keep the mind disturbed. Therefore, you should make sure that the place you choose to sleep in is calm and you create a peaceful environment in which you can enjoy deep sleep.

How does blue light affect our sleep?

The blue light emitted by our devices, badly affect our sleep. It strengthens the brain waves which increase alertness and suppress the sleep-inducing waves. By keeping your phone close to you, the emissions of radiation can be harmful and hazardous to your bodily functions. Your inability to have deep restful sleep affects your mood and performance at work. Therefore it is advisable to switch off devices at least 30 minutes before going to bed. Turn off the Wi-Fi and put your phone further away from you.

In addition to a peaceful environment, meditation can be beneficial in providing you with good quality sleep. It is advisable to go to bed in a peaceful environment, with positive thoughts, being grateful for whatever was the outcome of the day. Gratitude and positive visualisation when retiring to bed will drift your mind into a resting state.

CHAPTER 11

TAP IN TO YOUR INNERSELF

It is essential to connect to yourself and be aware of what you are capable of. You might have no idea about your hidden powers, but if you want to make the most out of your life, you must tap into your inner self and recognize your real worth. Once you know who you are, you can strive in the right direction to get what pleases you instead of chasing what others want for you.

You have to be yourself, set your own goals and do what you desire to do. Here are a few things that can help you to gain more confidence by making you realise what you really are and what you actually want.

Self-talk is important

When it comes to achieving something big or small in life, self-talk is one of the most important things. It leaves a substantial impact on your self-image and esteem. Most importantly, good self-talk can boost your confidence, and make you feel good about yourself. It is fundamentally important that you pay attention to your inner dialogue.

Development of a new mindset

The way you think about yourself and the world including everything in it can play a significant role in making you happy or unhappy, content or dissatisfied, grateful or thankless and calm or anxious. Your quality of life is in your hands. You can keep yourself motivated by creating an internal shift which can transform your personality. If you want to become a better version of yourself, you must develop a new mindset and let your inner self grow to start a new beginning.

The role of affirmations

Positivity is one of the major contributing factors to make you happy and content. The self-affirmations play a significant role in providing you with positive energy. By repeating the affirmations, you can train your mind to stay positive, and it can bring amazing consequences.
For instance, you can begin with using one affirmation daily to keep yourself motivated. You can make your own affirmations.

Here are some of the helpful affirmations that you can use.

- I am my own boss.
- I can do whatever I want.
- I am enthusiastic and energetic.
- I am peaceful and calm.
- I am free from all tension.
- I can fulfill my dreams.
- My mind is in my control.
- I can control my feelings.
- I am happy with myself.
- I am going to persevere regardless.

Spend some quality time with yourself

No matter how busy you are, it is essential that you take some time out for yourself and enjoy some 'Me-Time'. Disconnect yourself from the outside world, sit in silence and connect with your divine self. Talk to yourself, listen to your inner thoughts, and make it a routine to have this time with your inner self for at least 10 minutes.

Become teachable and receptive

If you want to improve yourself and gain success in life, you must have a receptive mind and a teachable spirit. You might not know whether you are teachable or not. But you can definitely make efforts to keep your teachability index high. Surround yourself with inspiring people, learn from them and remember that there is always room for improvement.

Get closer to nature

Nature is your best friend. The closer you get to it, the more peaceful you will be. Make it a routine to go for a walk daily and spend some time alone. Switch off your devices including phone and tablets and observe your surroundings. Look at the sky, trees, birds and listen to the silence of nature.

Hire a coach

The entire process of self-development can be very hectic. It can make you feel exhausted if you try without proper guidance. Googling tips from the internet is not the solution. You must seek professional help and hire a mentor. He will guide you throughout every step and make things comfortable for you.

Create new habits

With the help of a coach, you can reprogram your brain, create new thoughts, and thus create new and helpful habits that can contribute to the positive development of your personality.

BELIEFS WHEN CREATED TRIGGER RESPONSES FROM YOUR BRAIN WHICH DICTATE ATTITUDE.

CHAPTER 12

DARE TO DREAM

Your thoughts create your reality

If you want to achieve big, you must think big. Never underestimate yourself and be optimistic no matter how hard life seems to be. You might have no idea of your hidden potential. Your mind and your thoughts can shape your reality. Remember that everything happening in the physical world has an origin, a cause that is associated with your mental world.

Follow your dreams and have unshakeable Faith

By controlling your thoughts, you can control what happens in your life. You can create your own reality by using the power of your mind. You must believe in yourself and make the best of your efforts to achieve your dreams.

You might have heard the famous Martin Luther Kings Speech called 'I have a dream', in which he demonstrated his belief in his dream. In addition to Martin Luther who had a staunch belief in his dreams, several other known names also gained success by believing in their thoughts. You can take motivation from successful people who attained what they wanted only because they had unshakeable faith in their dreams. For instance, Mahatma Gandhi of India, the founder of Microsoft Bill Gates, the inventors of the aeroplane (the Wright brothers), and the 35th US president, John F. Kennedy (you must read his speech 'We choose to go to the moon'). These are some of the inspiring personalities who teach us to believe in ourselves. Their efforts are proof that perseverance pays off.

It is your tenacity, persistence and efforts that make your dreams come true. You always have a chance to attain success as long as you try for it. If you don't give up, you will definitely get what you desire.

I know I could do it

This attitude can lead you to success. Just believe in yourself, and you can achieve what you desire. It is evident that your attitude towards life affects the outcomes. For instance, the famous Athlete Dr Roger Bannister set an incredible record of running a mile under just four minutes. He made it possible by his passion and the power of belief in his dream. Just like him you can also attain whatever you want. With sheer dedication the impossible can become possible.

So what's stopping you?

All you need is perseverance, dedication and sincere efforts for the realisation of your dream. No matter how tough the circumstances are, you can go through them only if you stay put. So, what is stopping you from achieving your goals? Move ahead, stay determined, and nothing can prevent you from achieving success.

How do we achieve our dreams?

The power of repetition through visualisation

Here is a useful tip for making something happen. If you want to control what happens next in your life, you need to strengthen your imagination. Your visualisation techniques and using repetition to remind yourself that you can do this can be really helpful. By repetition through visualisation, you can make your mind believe that you can achieve your goals.

Accountability

In addition to imagination, self-accountability is also a beneficial way of keeping yourself motivated. Be honest and make sure that you are accountable to yourself.

Timeline

Scheduling is essential. If you want to achieve something big, you must make a plan. Design several steps for attaining short-term goals that can lead to your long-term goals. Make a timeline, create a to-do list and keep monitoring your progress after regular intervals.

Celebration and Gratitude

Your constant efforts can bring forth positive outcomes. Don't be hard on yourself and acknowledge the little achievements as well to stay encouraged for the bigger goal. Celebrate little moments of success by praising yourself. Your gratitude and self-appreciation can pave your way towards long-term success.

SUPERCHARGE, INSPIRE, ENERGISE AND MOTIVATE THE SUBSCONSCIOUS MIND.

CHAPTER 13
THE 5 C'S TO HEALING

The healing process works to take the diseased, damaged and unbalanced organism back a state of health through detox and rebuilding. Different techniques can be applied to help someone to heal from small, all the way to critical damage.

The 5 C's to healing are as follows:

1. Choice

The ability to heal is in God's grasp. Yet, the decision to be healed is yours. Everybody, in some dimension, needs healing. You may have petitioned God for healing ordinarily for a long time. Maybe you have lived with your brokenness so long that you have become used to it. Perhaps you ponder exactly when God will take all the hurt away. He can. In any case, you likewise should release the hurt and let the healing start.

Making the necessary correct life changing decisions to overcome our personal problems and fulfill our potential implies dismissing the falsehoods we regularly continue to buy into.
The decisions you make shape the adventure he wants for you.

He can and will heal you. Be that as it may, you should put

one foot before the other and let go and allow him to do his work. His word certifies that God needs us to encounter His healing, yet we usually settle on decisions that hinder this encounter towards transformation.

When we glance back at how the past turns and bends in the pathways of our lives, we can see critical decisions we made, which made the lives we have now. It furnishes us with a guide for settling on the correct choices today to give us a better way to tomorrow.

I am requesting that you surrender your life as you are aware of it so you can discover the existence God has for you. Grab hold of your future today and settle on the decisions that will prompt your healing. Participate during the time spent healing, and experience passionate and otherworldly experiences, and in some cases physical healing. Change brokenness into your new life mission. Distinguish the enormous falsehoods that forestall you in encountering passionate, profound, and physical healing.

2. Chance

We should give a chance for our body and mind to heal itself. The formula of healing ourselves is buried deep inside us. Relaxation, rest and meditation can help our body have a better chance to heal.

Meditation is a constant process of preparing your psyche to center and divert your thoughts. You can utilise it to build familiarity with yourself and your environment. Numerous individuals consider it an approach to decrease pressure and create focus. Numerous styles of meditation can help diminish pressure.

Meditation can likewise lessen side effects in individuals with stress-activated medical conditions. A few types of

Meditation can reduce sadness and cultivate an increasingly uplifting point of view. Research demonstrates that keeping up a continuous propensity for meditation may enable you to maintain these states of mind.

The benefits of standard meditation are that it helps to build memory and mental lucidity, and can deter age related memory loss and dementia. Meditation can also lessen the perception of pain in the mind. This may help treat interminable pain when utilized as an enhancement to medical care or exercise based therapy.

3. Change

By the day's end, Change creates opportunity. The issue is in our disposition towards Change, regardless of whether we treat it adversely or we invite it and acknowledge it. Given the way that change is, in that it is the normal condition of things and is inescapable, you have two options: you can grasp Change, or you can dismiss it. Consider the upside of inescapable change and take your chances. Give change a chance to end up as an appreciated ordeal for yourself and your body. We all realize that nothing will be enhanced without anyone else. We have to do things any other way to get that going. Without Change, there'd be no upgrades and improvements.

Changes trigger advancement. Things push ahead and are created due to the change. Changing our thoughts will move us close to healing our body and mind. Negative thoughts block the way of healing. It does nothing but increase our tension and pain physically and emotionally. Thinking of good things can change our behavior towards different things and gives a chance for our body to heal itself. We can increase the chances of getting healed by just changing our mood towards it. Thinking positive towards it all will help you to heal mentally, and the body will detect these good thoughts and increase chances of physical healing. It will also help us to relieve some pain and stress. And in the process of time we will know that it is helping us to heal from the illness.

4. Confidence

Self-confidence is viewed as one of the most crucial and compelling helpers and controllers of conduct in one's regular daily existence. Self-confidence is certainly not a persuasive point by itself. It is a judgment about abilities for achievement of some objective, and, consequently, must be considered inside a more extensive conceptualization of inspiration that gives your objectives context.

Confidence can assist you with taking on the world with more vitality and assurance, bringing about better connections, quality work and a sentiment of being associated with your environment. Self-confident individuals, as a rule, can impact others much more effortlessly, and in addition, control their own feelings and practices all the more mindfully.

5. Continuity

Continuity of care is all about embracing a considerate attitude towards treatment and it lessens the dangers of pointless testing and the potential for medicinal blunders. Your provider definitely knows your past therapeutic and individual history and in addition the conditions of your day to day life. Along these lines, any choices made should be the best ones for you. Continuity of care is one of the main and necessary elements to achieve healing. Healing with constant care and medication along with consistent methods can increase the chance of healing the body and mind and provides better results over time.

Meditation

Connecting with your mind through meditation in the early hours of the morning or any time through the day can have a noticeable impact on your wellbeing. By breathing deeply through your nose and exhaling through the mouth this can help shift toxic gases and create more oxygen in our brains. Focusing on the solar chakra which is your belly button can help release blockages and bring and generate more peace and creativity in the unconscious mind. You can generate powerful, positive thoughts and visualizations in your mind which brings the positive influence of peace and serenity to your facial muscles.

The benefits of meditation help reduce stress and this inadvertently helps us control our anxiety, and promotes emotional health. Regular practice of meditation relaxes us, and deep breathing creates many powerful physiological changes. Listening to harmonious peaceful music in deep meditation helps relax the muscles and all your worries, and can aid in fighting various diseases and alter the structure of our DNA.

Gratitude

We have to thank God for what we have now; to be able to be present and think about the blessed times to come.
Be grateful for what you have achieved so far and ask for strength to achieve more in the future. Through meditation you must relax all your muscles and be able to feel the surge of activity within your body and maintain your breathing at the same time.

Visualisation

Imagine things are happening to you i.e. having money, getting a new job etc. You need to think positively about what's in your life and what's new that you want to achieve. Make an imaginary story of what you want to achieve that will make you happy. It's like looking ahead about things that will bring you success and healthy relationships with friends and family.

The best things in life will come if we think about them through our feelings and act from that inspiration, even visualizing yourself by sitting by the beach or something that makes you feel happy, can create a more harmonious and peaceful life. Attract positivity and not negativity because the best things in life will come when we imagine exactly what we want and when we work to achieve it.

Following your dreams – You have the power to achieve if you act with passion and determination. Whatever you want in life, draw a picture in your mind because the universe is there to give you what you desire. You will attract the right things if you start taking action and with the spirit of your mindset you'll be able to achieve those goals be it good health, wealth or prosperity in your career. Action takers and go getters make their dreams come true. Things will happen in life sometimes when you least expect them. Because you've put positive thoughts in your subconscious mind you will be able to implement them and open door ways to new opportunities and a better life. Dreams are not only for dreamers but also those who will practice through the relaxation medium and through their subconscious mind

Words of Martin Luther King

"I have a dream that one day this nation will rise up and live out the true meaning of its creed - we hold these truths to be self-evident: that all men are created equal." "Let us not seek to satisfy our thirst for freedom by drinking from the cup of bitterness and hatred."

CHAPTER 14
DIFFERENT THERAPIES AND THEIR BENEFITS

With decades of clinical experience in alternative and holistic medicine, I have undertaken various methods and practices as part of the recovery process for my patients. In this chapter I will be discussing in detail the different types of therapies which I administer along with their benefits.

Background in Alternative & Holistic Medicines

Holistic medicine treats the whole person and not just their symptoms, and in my practice I also help to rectify the social blockages to get the patient's life back on track.

When the patient is stuck and rigid, the shift will happen when they look at the State and Situation, when we realise it's stuck in either their core values or having a conflict in their mind.

Those medicines that are used in place of conventional or experimental medicines are known as alternative medicines. These medicines are usually unproven, sometimes harmful, and ineffective in some cases. When we talk about Wholistic (holistic) medicines, it means those medicines are used to heal the whole person. Here, the whole person means that they are used to heal emotions, body, mind, and spirit of a person. A holistic therapist believes that our body is a system of connected parts and if one part is in pain, the other will suffer too. Different types of treatments are used with alternative and holistic medicines to treat people.

Benefits:
- These medicines work for the prevention of diseases.
- You will get personal attention.
- They help to change the way one thinks about different subjects.

Colon Hydrotherapy

As we all know, a toxic stool can lead to severe pain and health issues for a person. In a colonic irrigation the colon is thoroughly cleansed using warm water to remove the solid or toxic stool, gas or related waste. The water is injected into the rectum in a suitably safe manner. This therapy is entirely effective as well as relaxing for a person suffering through this issue. The best thing about colon hydrotherapy is that no chemicals and drugs are used in the overall process which ensures it is a safe treatment for everyone.

Benefits:
- Colon hydrotherapy is very effective in building a strong immune system.
- It helps prevent constipation because constipation is the root cause of many other diseases.
- It helps our body to increase the absorption of minerals and vitamins in the bloodstream.
- Increases energy
- Reduces bloatedness, fluctuance and belching
- Improves digestion as the stagnated faecal pathway is cleared and with repeat treatment nutrient absorption is improved.
- Furthermore with bowel regularity after colonics and softer stools the likelihood of hemorrhoids and piles is lessened

- Improved alertness, concentration and clarity with enhanced quality and better overall functionality for the patient.

The benefits are numerous and can vary from patient to patient and unwanted bacteria and food can be a toxin to the body and an overload to the lower abdomen causing discomfort. Probiotics are suggested to patients to balance the Flora bacteria in the gut.

In the two decades of my practice as a Colon Hydro therapist, all patients showed great positive relief from their symptoms and improved considerably, with feelings of lightness and reduced symptoms of lower abdominal distention.

Case study 1:
A 38 year old patient came to my clinic with symptoms of indigestion, bloatedness, heartburn and he was also suffering from acid reflux. Having evaluated his hectic city life and erratic eating habits, I also looked at his past and present situation and the state of why he was so uncomfortable. We unraveled and found he had gone through the trauma of childhood bullying and low marks in school exams that lead him into a rushed and trapped state of mind. And as soon as I dealt with his letting go of his past, the tension in his muscles and lower colon was much reduced. He was more relaxed and we achieved more success with repeat colonics, and with suggested herbs for digestion used for relining the osepohaghal wall, and he was free from 15 years of suffering.

Case study 2:
A 40 year old female patient suffered from very uncomfortable bloated feelings and after assessing her diet, we gave her a diet plan with repeat colonics and she showed great improvement with herbal remedies for bowel and digestion. And more over colonics also helped the circulation

in her legs and that helped reduce the swelling in her ankles.

Naturopathy

Naturopathy involves the natural healing powers of an individual's body. The main focus of naturopathy is on the factors that are causing the disease. Unlike other therapies, it does not focus on treating the symptoms of a certain disease in a person. In naturopathy, when the action is performed on the causes of a disease, the body becomes able to fight against a disease or to heal. Thus, it can be stated that the naturopathy is performed in those cases where we need to restore the vital functions of a person's body.

Benefits:
Naturopathy helps to cure many diseases like:
- Obesity
- Digestive problems
- Infertility issues
- Chronic pain
- Hormonal issues
- Allergies
- Headaches

Case study:
A 49 year female with 15 years of headaches and depression and body aches and pains was treated with a combination of practices: nutritional therapies, Ayurveda herbal remedies and acupuncture. After assessment in her second session there was marked improvement with her symptoms. She slept for 10 hours without a break in her sleep and over the next few months she experienced healing in her other symptoms, and the state of her health improved remarkably.

Herbal/ Ayurveda Remedies

The sources from where herbal remedies come from is an

important factor. Whether they are organically farmed, the condition of soil, climate, and how they are dried and stored all determine the quality.

The quality and potency of herbs is important to consider. When taking herbal remedies one is getting close to nature as these are in concentrate extract form, powder form and liquid form (in different potencies). They are also created for teas, and they also come fresh or in the form of dried plant roots or leaves. Some of the herbs and seeds we use in cooking have beneficial properties.

Herbal remedies are given after assessment, taking into consideration the allopathic drugs patient has been prescribed.

Benefits:
- The main advantage of using herbal medicines is to improve one's health and maintain it through these dietary supplements.
- These medicines help to boost the immune system.
- They work best to maintain balanced hormone levels.

Case study:
Over the years, my patients have recovered from a whole host of conditions with my range of Ayurveda/ herbal remedies.

A particular patient of mine, a young mother who was breast feeding her baby, developed eczema (dermatitis skin condition). After assessment she was prescribed with body soap, creams and lotions for hydrating the skin and with anti-itch drops.

Dedication from the mother in applying the creams and hydrating her skin over the next few months cleared the eczema. But in assessment it was noted that the sugar content in her desserts that the mother was eating was one of the causes of her skin flare up.

So cutting out all hidden sugars helped in her recovery process too.

Aromatherapy

Aromatherapy is a massage that is done using different aromatic oils. Smell is the most active sense, so the aromatic oils have wonderful effects on body and mind.
Massage in aromatherapy has healing and calming effects to the body and skin. Also, aromatherapy is considered both a science and an art, and it is gaining popularity in the field of medicine.

Benefits:
• Aromatic oils help to calm the emotions and mind.
• Essential oils help to uplift your mood and overall health.
• They provide relief from inflammation and pain.

Case study:
A gentleman working in a stressful medical environment was suffering from anxiety and insomnia. We worked with a combination of Aromatherapy oils with base oils. With three treatments and relaxation massage his sleep was much improved and he was coping, with more confidence. Moreover his anxiety attacks were much better with Ayurveda and nutritional remedies.

Lymphatic Massage

Lymphatic massage is also known by other names such as manual lymph drainage and lymphatic drainage. This type of massage is a very useful technique to release fluid from the body. Sometimes after major surgery or operations, your body may have stagnated fluid in the lymph nodes, and most doctors recommend lymphatic massage to their patients to release the waste from their body.

Benefits:
- Lymphatic massage helps women to reduce their breast soreness and help in feeding their little one.
- It helps to boost the body's immune system.
- It also relaxes the body because it helps to reduce pain.
- Helps to reduce inflammation
- Rapidly speeds up the removal of toxins from the lymphatic system
- Encourages natural drainage of the lymph from the body tissue

Case study:

A 55 year old gentleman with chronic edema in his legs had regular lymphatic drainage in a structured way to help shift the water retention in his legs. It also involved a complete lifestyle and dietary change with suggestion of elevating his legs above his heart level whilst resting. It involved intake of water throughout the day which helped open the bladder and clean up the stagnated toxins from the lymphatic system.

Reflexology

Reflexology is generally called a tension and stress reliever. Reflexology uses a special technique in which the therapist applies pressure on the feet and hands by using a special finger and thumb technique. It focuses on the reflex areas of the body that need to relax.

Benefits:
- The most important advantage of reflexology is that it gives relaxation from pain.
- It helps to improve nerve and brain functions.
- It increases the blood circulation in the human body.
- It helps to boost energy levels.

- It can relieve menstrual cramps.

NES Energetic WellNES scan/ NES BioEnergetiX WellNES System

The NES energetic wellness scan is a unique technique to help experts to restore a client's health using three steps, i.e. assess, rejuvenate, and re-imprint.

NES health scan can be used:

- to address body field issues concerning physical, emotional and mental states.
- As part of the ongoing daily health and exercise program.
- To enhance other complementary health therapies

The complete NES program works at a deep, holistic level connecting the state of your body-field with your body's own innate self-healing intelligence. NES provides a natural and non-invasive way to foster positive changes in the state of your overall well-being.

After the scan, liquid preparations are given according to the readings that show distress on the organ, on the state of mind and body. Each of these infoceuticals are formulated and coded with information to correct the specific body fields. The added advantage is that the infoceuticals are compatible with herbal supplements, pharmaceutical medicines or other remedies you may be taking.

Benefits:
- It is very helpful in restoring the health and energy of a human body.
- **Improves Emotional resiliency**
  - ➢ where you cope better with stress and life challenges

➢ where you have the ability to go with the flow and relax with certain situations
- **Increases vitality and energy**
  ➢ More stamina
  ➢ Improved sleep
  ➢ Sharper mental focus
  ➢ Increased drive and motivation
- **Physical or emotional issues**
  ➢ Relief from or improvements to physical or emotional issues

Case study:

The parents of a very critically ill ten year old child with a colitis condition were given little hope of recovery other than a surgical procedure of a colostomy. After assessment and having done the NES scan and the protocol of Ayurveda remedies, with powders to help with the inflammation in the gut wall, we also complemented this treatment with the NES infoceuticals. The parents practiced the protocol suggested on the child. Within a few days they showed no blood stools and their digestion improved and their cramps and pains reduced in their lower abdomen. Assessments and treatments over the next few months helped the patient to recover fully from the inflammation of their colon and to the parent's relief and joy; their child did not have to undergo any surgical intervention.

Diet & Nutrition

Going back to before fire was discovered, to the stone age, to Industrialization, mankind's food and diet has evolved and as our foods get more processed with preservatives, the value of the food we ingest decreases.

Diet and good nutrition is very important to support our body to fight against multiple diseases.

A healthy diet should include fruits, vegetables, whole grains, protein grains such as Quinoa, cous cous, millet, wholegrain bread, brown pasta, fresh noodles, a variety of nuts, low fat dairy products, legumes, a variety of beans, nuts, eggs and if you are non-vegetarian, a variety of lean meats, fish, poultry and eggs.

Eating a variety of foods helps with maintaining good health and provides a range of different nutrients to the body.
Good wholesome nutrition also reduces the risk of disease and protects the organs. A balanced diet and nutrition is vital for our organs and tissues, to repair the wear and tear of our muscles, and it increases our physical and mental performance. It is through food we get fuel which converts to energy.

Benefits:

- it helps the human body to maintain and achieve overall balance and keep fit
- It helps heart disease, cholesterol, bone disease, blood pressure, and joints.
- Maintains our immune system, which protects from illnesses
- Eating healthy can positively affect our mood
- Increase focus
- Increase life expectancy
- Can delay ageing.

Case study:

A 30 year old female with a hectic family lifestyle was assessed and due to the swelling in her feet and ankles and being obese at the time we offered her a diet plan, where we cut out all hidden sugars and supported her diet with essential herbs. As she had very poor circulation, after six treatments of reflexology working with different areas of her feet, she began to notice her feet were not as cold and the water retention in her feet improved over the weeks. But we had to encourage her to walk, when she increased her water intake, and with her dietary changes she became more confident when she began to lose weight.

Definition of a Reiki master

Reiki is an effective Japanese technique that is used to heal mental and physical illness. In Reiki, 'rei' means higher intelligence and 'ki' means non-physical energy. Using the Reiki technique of placing hands on the areas of concern, effectively the therapist can channel energy into that area through the heat of their hands. It is an art of spiritual healing. Reiki master needs special training to become a master, but it is not compulsory to affiliate with any religious authority. Reiki is not a new technique and it has been known since 1922. Reiki techniques include infusion, centering, beaming, clearing and so on.

Benefits:
- It provides relaxation to those who are facing stress and anxiety.
- It helps to cure infertility and heart disease.
- It heals you mentally and emotionally.
- Can help to reduce pain.
- Patients will feel refreshed and may even fall asleep during the session
- Can give relief from headaches
- Helps patient with clarity, shifting negative emotions
- A general sense of wellbeing

Case study:
A 55 year old patient suffered from regular headaches and impaired sleep. Channeling Reiki was relaxing and she coped better in her daily routine and office environment.

Juicing

The benefits of juicing are numerous. I create a juice diet for my patients depending on the condition they are suffering from. Every Vegetable and fruit has some healing properties hence the right kinds of juices are advised depending on your body type. With a quality masticating Juicer you will be retaining more nutrients compared to centrifugal juicing which spins the fruit and vegetable out at speed. There is more fiber in juice that has been extracted with a centrifugal juicer.

Benefits:
- full of nutrients and fiber
- cleanses
- detoxes
- stops hunger
- good for bowel regularity
- thirst quencher

Case study:
All patients have given a positive feedback upon consuming juice. The correct combination of juice is advised per patient, depending on their symptoms. There is more fiber in juice that has been extracted with a mascating juicer.

Acupuncture

Acupuncture is a Traditional Chinese Medicine going back 2,500 years and it involves the insertion of fine needles into the skin at specific points (meridian lines). As the needles are inserted to various depths it increases the flow of Qi energy throughout the body. By restoring the balance of energy it alleviates pain and improves general health. Acupuncture has numerous benefits.

Benefits:
- Knee pain
- Neck pain
- Lower back pain

- Migraines and headache
- Osteoarthritis
- Morning sickness
- Painful periods
- Emotional disorders
- Digestive disorders
- Fibromyalgia
- Asthma

Case study:

A 38 year old female in a teaching profession suffered from acute lower back pain which was impairing her movement whilst teaching. After assessment and offering her three Acupuncture treatments, she improved and had no pain that she had previously suffered from for four years. She also had three Ayurveda massages to reduce the tension in her upper back.

Ayurveda

Ayurveda is the old massage therapy, which is called the science of life. The meaning is derived from the therapy name Ayur "life," and Veda "science." Ayurveda therapy is based on two principles: the first is that mind and body are connected; the second is that nothing can heal and transform better than the power your mind.

Benefits:

- Ayurveda is great therapy to reduce stress.
- It plays a crucial part in establishing the hormonal balance
- Ayurveda healing techniques help to reduce inflammation.
- It boosts up the body functions and maintains overall balance.

Case study:
The use of different combinations of hot Ayurveda oils with lymphatic drainage, and the use of heat pouches in Potli massage has helped to relieve pain, and improve flexibility and blood circulation in my patients. They have felt rejuvenated, relaxed, and felt more flexible in areas of their body that they previously experienced stiffness in. Using this old age technique has given relief to patients with osteoarthritis, spinal arthritis, rheumatoid arthritis and joint inflammation, naming only a few. Potli massage also helps to stimulate blood circulation and gives you healthier looking skin. The heated oils open up pores and relaxes the muscles, providing a therapeutic effect by nourishing, rejuvenating and improving general blood circulation.

Each Potli massage is done with different techniques to suit he patient's symptoms and tailored to each individual.

Ayurveda herbs in liquid form

Ayurveda is an ancient medicine closest to nature and has been practiced for over 5,000 years. I have a range of niche Ayurveda formulations to assist in a whole host of illnesses. The imbalances in one of the three bodily energies of pitta, vatta and kapha can make a person more susceptible to disease.

The liquid formulations are created according to the patient's symptoms and help the body to heal. Disturbances in any one of the doshas are addressed with Ayurveda herbal remedies in various doses according to patients and the modality of the disease.

Ayurveda can help to treat inflammation, digestive and hormonal imbalances and infertility. Extracts in liquid, powder or capsules also benefit the conditions listed below, naming only a few.

Benefits:
- can help with painful menstruation
- liver/ kidney detox
- high blood pressure
- cholesterol
- balancing blood sugars
- memory
- urinary tract
- asthma
- hay fever
- boosting immune system
- anxiety
- depression
- joint pains
- skin conditions/eczema/ psoriasis/ skin dermatitis
- sinus conditions
- digestive disorders
- migraines
- fatigue
- boosts energy
- intestinal parasites
- heart burn/ belching

Case study:

A 21 year old university student took a break from his university course because the inflammation of his skin on his face, body and lips was keeping him awake at night and disrupting his concentration at university. He took time off and became very anti-social because of his condition.

When the patient came for assessment we looked at all the symptoms and after a NES scan also diagnosed him with a fungal skin condition. Appropriate Ayurveda remedies, lotions, creams and potions were given to assist in healing in his skin dermatitis condition which was borderline psoriasis as well. Having implemented a diet and lifestyle change the patient showed rapid transformation in his skin texture in one month and noticed a reduction in inflammation and began to have rested sleep. His skin improved remarkably without flaking and the scarring and discolouration of the skin was the last stage I dealt with. The patient has now completed his university degree and has continued to implement the same diet that was suggested.

DIVE INTO THE SEA OF GRATITUDE, YOU WILL SEE YOURSELF AS A WINNER.

ABOUT THE AUTHOR

$\mathbf{D}$r. Manjit Kaur was born in Kenya and continued her further studies in the UK and four other continents in Holistic Medicine. She is now a skilled and qualified practitioner in eleven therapies, and has helped thousands of patients recover from a whole host of symptoms and life threatening illnesses when the NHS had given no hope for patients other than surgery or chemo.

Dr Manjit Kaur has also been very successful in helping couples to conceive with 90% success for women with polycystic ovaries syndrome (PCOS) or history of infertility in both males and females.

Renowned worldwide in Asian Media, she has hosted Radio and TV shows for over 20 years and has hosted four TV shows per week on SKY. The health shows that she has appeared on are cook shows (vegetarian cooking) and chat shows (talking about community related issues).

She is also a philanthropist, public speaker, TV presenter, coach, and award winner of the Sikh Sewadar for community work.

With charity very close to Dr. Manjit Kaur's heart, she has put large funds into a mammoth water irrigation project with the Bantu tribe in Meru, Kenya. Dr. Manjit Kaur continued to set up an Agave plant in Soroti in Uganda. She has worked with and helped widows in Punjab to open small businesses and she has guided and coached patients in drug addiction centers, also in Punjab.

Dr Manjit Kaur has a tireless, bouncing, energetic,

charismatic personality, and she aims to empower all her clients with the will to Achieve, with enthusiasm and continued perseverance.

Dr. Manjit Kaur does not know how to give up. She presses on until the goal is achieved. Her smile is her strength and her experience you will embrace. Her persistence in reaching her goals will magnetise and encourage you.

She has spent her life attaining knowledge of holistic and natural medicine. After running five clinics over two decades, she is now inspiring, training, coaching, and teaching the general public, practitioners and entrepreneurs on how to live and achieve a more balanced harmonious life through the application of a healthy lifestyle. She walked alone to find her path, and took challenges in countries and places where no women would dare to go. Her passion, her strength, her ability, her dreams, her patience, and her endurance to survive the roughest terrains is the making of her "Blueprint".

Let's join hands together to make

"YOUR HEALTH, YOUR WEALTH"

Dr. Manjit Kaur is a Holistic Practitioner of Alternative Medicines & Naturopathy. She is well renowned around the globe for her radio, national & satellite T.V for health and cook shows shown on the Sikh channel and Akaal channel on SKY and YouTube. Dr. Manjit is well qualified and equipped with decades of clinical experiences. She practices Alternative & Wholistic (also pronounced Holistic) Medicines, which includes Colon Hydrotherapy, Naturopathy, Herbal Medicines, Aromatherapy, Lymphatic Massage, Reflexology, NES BioEnergetiX WellNES System, Diet & Nutrition, and she is also a Reiki master.

She is certified in Acupuncture, Ayurveda & Panchkarma from D.A.V College, Jalandhar, India. She has held free Ayurveda & Acupuncture treatment camps in India and Italy and treated patients suffering from long term illnesses.

Modern allopathic science addresses problems at a different level, but in holistic medicines she treats patients by balancing their mental, physical and spiritual state. She believes healing is a process which requires not only particular medicines, but a spiritual connection with complete devotion from the patient including committing in making long lasting lifestyle and dietary change. She establishes a trust based bond with patients, slowly unravelling the root causes of diseases and uncovers how it manifested emotionally, to understand how it caused additional physical or mental problems. She has brought awareness to many with her knowledge on healthy nutrition and how proper diet enhances the body's efficiency. She provides unlimited mentoring and support to her patients, as she believes this is key for the patient's successful recovery. A balanced diet is the key to rejuvenation. An equilibrium and balance between body, mind and spirit is the key to a blissful life. She has cured patients which according to modern science were impossible to heal.

Dr. Manjit is also training students on how to become good practitioners and how to make more accurate clinical observations in order to get the best results. Besides Mentoring Dr. Manjit is now also doing National Stage Shows with her unique branded system (UBS) and does Mastermind classes for groups to learn about the 5 steps she has created.

At her Vitality and Rejuvenation Clinics you can achieve major changes in your health.

Dr. Manjit believes without a doubt there is a connection between health, the mind, the body and the spirit. Disease steps in when there is an emotional imbalance, then physical problems surface, syndromes such as fatigue, allergies, hormonal imbalances, toxic overload, organ and structural imbalance, vitamin and mineral deficiencies to mention a few. Feel clean inside and outside with Colon Hydrotherapy combined with other therapies.

This book will take you on the journey of self-discovery and realization on how to have a healthier and wealthier lifestyle through her unique Body Balance Blueprint^{TM} which was created around her Unique Branded System.

TESTIMONIALS

Trilight treatment

The infection and abscesses on both my feet in Dec 2017 led to deep tissue infection which further led to gangrene. I lost all feeling on my feet and skin. I was admitted to hospital in January 2018 with serious grade 4 infection and my feet were heavily bandaged due to 9 pockets of pus and weeping wounds on both feet. My work was seriously jeopardised due to the two month admission. Numerous anti-inflammatory drugs and antibiotics were administered intravenously but my infection was not reducing. I was given the serious life changing option of amputation. My feet were plastered for six months.

If my wife had not approached you to come to hospital to see what other options I could have other than amputation, today my disability would have further changed my daily movements. Dr Manjit, your Trilight treatment was a life saviour for me. Two and a half days with 16 Trilight treatments, which you administered at my home, helped me achieve recovery. I had no more weeping wounds. I could put weight on my feet without the wounds seeping pus. Miraculously as per your observation I had new skin collagen and tissue repair. We took your instructions and cancelled routine hospital/nurse appointments to bandage the wounds. Ten days later I walked back to hospital without any bandages.

To the shock of Doctors and nurses and their observations I did not need amputation or plastering. Dr Manjit, as per your assurance I was back to work 3 weeks later.

Thank you for all you have done. You achieved results beyond the Doctors allopathic treatment. I realised life is so precious. I am celebrating a new life now. Thank you for your professionalism in alternative medicine. Your passion to achieve goals and assist me is commendable. Thanks a million.

~M.S

I was battling with acne for ten years from the age of 11. This affected my confidence a lot and I became very shy. I heard about Manjit Kaur's treatment on TV and after consultation preceded with Skin care treatments and remedies Followed by TRILIGHT treatments and masks and I am so pleased to say my acne scars and blemishes have improved by 90%. If I have the odd outbreak it heals very fast and I don't shy away now. Manjit looked into my diet a lot and helped me implement the right foods which were healthier for me. I want to thank Manjit for all she did.

~ S.K. (South London)

Chronic colitis

Time was against us and the odds were thin for our eight year old daughter's and her battle with Chronic Colitis

We pleaded with Doctors to discharge Aman for 8 hours from Hospital and to allow us to get her to Manjit Kaur who we were recommended to.

With four days left to having a full colostomy, she had inflammation of the colon and had ten blood stools a day. We went to Manjit with faith and after assessment and an NES SCAN, Aman's treatment was started and on the same night there was a dramatic change with only one stool showing minor bleeding and more improvement the following three days.

The surgery was cancelled and Doctors were very pleased with Aman's recovery.

Sixteen years on she has proceeded with her higher education and University with no problems.

We would like to thank Manjit for her support in giving Aman a new life.

~ **P. Kaur**

Digestive problems

Having had 20 years of digestive issues, my treatment and all the food support I received has improved my condition and I no longer have any digestion problems. I do eat all the foods that she recommended and now live a happier life

~ **Gurdev. W.Mid**

Fertility problems

I have been blessed with a beautiful baby.
Having struggled to conceive with allopathic methods and two IVF treatments which failed, and having lost twins at 23 weeks, I was told that I would never carry a baby to full term, as I was tested for a rare genetic disposition.

Having taken Dr. Manjit's advice and her herbal fertility protocol I conceived in two months and carried my baby to full term, with all her support in developing a positive mindset, diet and nutrition.

We have celebrated our son's first birthday and would like

to thank Dr. Manjit for all her support.

I also suffered with joint pains and having had treatment from Dr. Manjit Kaur it's great to be free from pain and not to live on four painkillers a day.

~ G K W Midlands

Having suffered from bloated feelings and indigestion for years, I went to see Manjit, having had a series of Colon hydrotherapy treatments. It was the best investment I did for my health.

~G.S (London)

Detox! Wow! Now that's what I call a Detox. I never knew I was carrying so much stagnated waste matter in spite of opening my bowels. I was always low on energy and having a feeling of fullness. Having had Colon hydrotherapy treatment I was shocked what was still in me. I got immediate relief and would recommend a quarterly Detox.

~Monica

NES "The BioEnergetiX WellNes System"

I had NES Scan and was totally blown away by the information that was picked up and related to my present situation. The infoceutical drops given to me shifted my blockages and in 48 hours I noticed a massive change in my energy and the pain in my knees were gone. I would come back for another Scan after finishing the drops.

~J.K

I had read about Energy medicine and booked a NES scan. I loved the accuracy of my diagnosis and was impressed with the effectiveness and there was a profound change in my health.

~B.S

I lived with stress & anxiety all the time and I had the NES scan and had a health treatment. (the Peace cycle session). Manjit also advised me to take Peace and Chill drops which has helped me tremendously to relax and sleep better

~G.B (West Midlands)

After my Colon Hydrotherapy session I was advised about food changes and my greatest energy surge came from the juices Manjit suggested. Oh what a difference Fresh juicing makes. The taste of Live juicing and the benefits have been so noticeable that I would not miss my AM juices as the kick start to my day.

~Dee

Colon hydrotherapy

I had a serious IBS condition which affected my daily routine. I was determined to get this IBS sorted and having had a series of Colon hydrotherapy sessions I am totally free from IBS symptoms and living a healthy vibrant life now and I am still juicing regularly.

~Rani (London)

Juicing was never in my diet but having met Manjit for a consultation for numerous digestive issues, I was really impressed with the advice. I started juicing which was advised for my symptoms and I have never looked back, as juicing has helped with digestive disorders and overcome the uncomfortable heartburn symptoms. With Manjit's Ayurveda remedies. I am living a healthier life now and still see Manjit for a regular body checkups and assessment.

~T.B (West Midlands)

I took four Ayurveda liquid complexes from Manjit after my consultation and noticed how my bowel regularity improved and I proceeded to do a Liver Cleanse with the Ayurveda herbs and I now have healthier digestion and no more burping, belching and no more bloated feelings. The Ayurveda complexes were not easy to take as they were quite bitter, but I am really pleased with the results.

~S Kaur

Book reviews

Dr Manjit Kaur's book is full of essential information and simple to follow guide for anyone who wants to have a healthy life and to avoid the Modern diseases which is seen in the News every day. It is based on years of her experience working with her clients and thousands of her audience in Radio and Television with great success.

~Philip Chan aka 10 Seconds Maths Expert,
   Award Winning Author and Radio Host,
   As seen on TV, Radio and Media

It has been a huge learning experience working on Doctor Manjit's book, and I thoroughly enjoyed it. The quality of the content is amazing, very comprehensive, clear and well laid out, and I have no doubt it will impact on thousands of people's lives.

~Laura Amherst, Book editor

This book entails a vast amount of information that will impact the lives of the readers. Dr. Manjit through her years of experience has shared with us her knowledge of how we could prevent diseases through alternative solutions rather than resorting to surgical and medical methods. The treatments which she has undertaken on her clients show clearly that her unique branded system works when implemented correctly. I thoroughly recommend this book to be read and for readers to get in contact with Dr Manjit if they really want to have a better lifestyle and health through alternative solutions.

~Labosshy Mayooran, Research Analyst, Author, Publisher & Mumpreneur

Dr. Manjit's book provides us with different therapies which can be implemented to prevent diseases. Through her life experiences and with the work she has undertaken with her clients she has put together a very informative book with the techniques that will help improve your health and lifestyle. I found the Trilight treatment to be very interesting to read about and was amazed by how that has helped so many of her clients. She has many YouTube videos of where she has broadcasted on TV in regards to how to overcome certain diseases which is something I highly recommend the readers to look in to. I'm sure this book will be very helpful and life changing for many.

~Mayooran Senthilmani, Finance Director, Author, Publisher & Inspirational and Empowerment Speaker

MESSAGE FROM THE AUTHOR

I hope after reading my book, whatever challenges you face in your life you can find the strength within you to get through everything. Reclaim your health through better self-awareness, life choices, dietary changes and exercise, staying connected with mother earth and nature.

Friends, life is a learning cycle, so keep your inner light lit and take control with positivity, keep ignited with compassion, and feel secure.

When you look after yourself and love the universe, it reflects on your communication with the people we are surrounded with and in our close relationships and our love has a rippling effect to others. I have explored chapters in this book of how our emotions affect our general wellbeing and how by taking control you reap the rewards of fulfillment, contentment and gratitude.

The Universe has a lot to give if you stay focused, calm and grateful in the present moment. Practicing visualisation and mindfulness exercises daily, you will be sowing seeds of harmony and positivity. By reading this book and implementing the guidance given about your health and wellbeing, you can begin changing your beliefs and perceptions, managing your stress, eating healthy foods, and sleeping soundly without taking your worries to bed. You will have a sense of peace.

With a balanced life applying the principles of self-adjustment, your body will function on an optimal level and you will celebrate youthfulness, vitality and wisdom.

It's never too late to set another goal, to recognize your ability to change and to create the healthier life you have always dreamt of!

~Dr Manjit Kaur

YouTube Videos

Injury & Collagen Repair Part 1
https://www.youtube.com/watch?v=7KJodyFmBoI

Trilight Treatment, Led, Acne, Injury & Collagen Repair Part 2
https://www.youtube.com/watch?v=Q4Yct892trs

Diabeties Part 1
https://www.youtube.com/watch?v=0q1fNXpVDfA

Diabeties Part 2
https://www.youtube.com/watch?v=j_v8k51YCiA

Fertility/ Infertility Part 1
https://www.youtube.com/watch?v=dU8XtV1WCAM

Fertility Part 2
https://www.youtube.com/watch?v=EIQT98ONB-o

Cupping Part 1
https://www.youtube.com/watch?v=h2d2Ag8_dxk

Cupping Part 2
https://www.youtube.com/watch?v=1wUfaWRDTEA

IBS, Constipation Part 1
https://www.youtube.com/watch?v=bLZNZadBSNQ

IBS, Constipation Part 2
https://www.youtube.com/watch?v=v0qCsAhVvqM

Gout, Raised Uric Acid Part 1
https://www.youtube.com/watch?v=EKtNhhE4lck

Gout, Raised Uric Acid Part 2
https://www.youtube.com/watch?v=cVxlw5LpRPs

Anti-Aging, Skin Radiance, Led Lights Part 1
https://www.youtube.com/watch?v=Fy4-ejUSEVM

Youthful Skin, Skin, Anti Aging, Collagen Part 2
https://www.youtube.com/watch?v=gOu7qKA-B4w

For more of my health videos please do subscribe to my YouTube channel "Dr Manjit Kaur" and healthy eating cookery shows on "akaalchannel".

www.ingramcontent.com/pod-product-compliance
Lightning Source LLC
Chambersburg PA
CBHW050128280326
41933CB00010B/1296